Workbook to Accompany

DENTAL ASSISTING

A Comprehensive Approach

Sixth Edition

T0198298

Workbook to Accompany

DENTAL ASSISTING

A Comprehensive Approach

Sixth Edition

Vaishali Singhal

Susan Kantz

Melissa Damatta

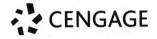

CENGAGE

Australia • Brazil • Canada • Mexico • Singapore • United Kingdom • United States

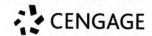

Workbook to Accompany Dental Assisting: A Comprehensive Approach, **6th Edition**
Vaishali Singhal, Susan Kantz, Melissa Damatta

SVP, Higher Education & Skills Product: Erin Joyner

VP, Higher Education & Skills Product: Thais Alencar

Product Director: Jason Fremder

Product Manager: Lauren Whalen

Product Assistant: Dallas Wilkes

Learning Designer: Mary Convertino

Senior Content Manager: Thomas Heffernan

Digital Delivery Lead: David O'Connor

Director, Marketing: Neena Bali

Marketing Manager: Courtney Cozzy

IP Analyst: Ashley Maynard

IP Project Manager: Kelli Besse

Production Service: Lumina Datamatics, Inc.

Designer: Felicia Bennett

Cover Image(s): istockphoto.com/XiXinXing

For product information and technology assistance, contact us at
Cengage Customer & Sales Support, 1-800-354-9706 or support.cengage.com.

For permission to use material from this text or product, submit all requests online at **www.cengage.com/permissions.**

Library of Congress Control Number: 2021914839

ISBN: 978-0-357-45665-1

Cengage
20 Channel Street
Boston, MA 02210
USA

Cengage is a leading provider of customized learning solutions with employees residing in nearly 40 different countries and sales in more than 125 countries around the world. Find your local representative at: **www.cengage.com.**

Cengage products are represented in Canada by Nelson Education, Ltd.

To learn more about Cengage platforms and services, register or access your online learning solution, or purchase materials for your course, visit **www.cengage.com.**

Printed at CLDPC, USA, 04-24

CONTENTS

Review of Textbook Chapters

Introduction

Introduction to the Dental Profession

SPECIFIC INSTRUCTIONAL OBJECTIVES

The student should strive to meet the following objectives and demonstrate an understanding of the facts and principles presented in this chapter:

1. Use terms presented in this chapter.
2. Identify the major milestones in dental history from ancient times to present day.
3. Name the individuals who had a great impact on the profession of dentistry.
4. Identify the people who promoted education and organized dentistry.
5. State the nine specialties of dentistry.
6. Describe career skills of the direct and indirect care dental team members.
7. List the education required for each dental career path.
8. List the professional organizations that represent each dental career path.
9. Explain the importance of being cross-trained.
10. Discuss the advances in dentistry.
11. Identify career opportunities for a dental assistant

VOCABULARY BUILDER

Matching

Match each term with the appropriate definition.

1. _____ analgesic
2. _____ calculus
3. _____ epidemiology
4. _____ extraoral

a. soft bacterial buildup

b. calcified buildup

c. part of oral mucous membranes

d. related to distribution of health-related events

4

5. _____ forensics

6. _____ gingiva

7. _____ oath

8. _____ plaque

9. _____ preceptorship

10. _____ prophylaxis

e. prevention of dental disease

f. promise

g. pain reliever

h. occurring outside of the oral cavity

i. supervision of a student by practicing professional

j. relating to application of science to legal issues

Fill in the Blank

Please fill in the blank with one of the choices provided.

prosthodontics a bridge	prosthodontics	dental sealant
dental dam	endodontics	prophylaxis
public health	a radiograph	orthodontics
pediatric dentistry	a prosthesis	the Bloodborne Pathogens Standard
periodontics	prosthodontics	

1. A _____ is a rubber sheet used to keep saliva from the teeth during dental procedures.

2. The resources and regulations that help to prevent health care workers from contracting infectious diseases are known as _____.

3. An artificial device that replaces a missing part from the body is known as _____.

4. The specialty that is involved in studying diseases that affect large populations is knows as _____.

5. The specialty that is involved in the diagnosis and treatment of children is known as _____.

6. The specialty that is involved in the straightening of teeth is known as _____.

7. The specialty that is involved in treating diseases pertaining to the area around the tooth is known as _____.

8. The specialty that is involved in the replacement of missing teeth is known as _____.

9. The specialty that is involved in treating diseases of the dental pulp is known as _____.

10. An image produced on film by the activation of x-ray radiation is known as _____.

CHAPTER REVIEW

True/False

Circle whether the answer is true of false.

1. **T**   **F**   Hippocrates discovered the x-ray.

2. **T**   **F**   Guy de Chauliac wrote the "Hygienic Rules for Oral Hygiene."

3. **T**   **F**   Robert Woofendale was one of the first dentists to arrive in the United States.

4. **T** **F** Josiah Flagg was the first dentist to use forensics.

5. **T** **F** Leonardo da Vinci was the first to distinguish between premolars and molars.

6. **T** **F** William Conrad Roentgen is known as the father of medicine.

7. **T** **F** John Baker was one of the dentists who treated George Washington.

8. **T** **F** Josiah Flagg was skilled in correcting cleft lip.

9. **T** **F** Hesi-Re is known for creating the dental chair with an extension arm for instruments.

10. **T** **F** Horace Hayden built a library of dental literature.

11. **T** **F** Public health is not a specialty of dentistry.

12. **T** **F** Dental hygiene programs may be 2 years or 4 years.

13. **T** **F** A licensed or registered dental hygienist can provide oral care education to their patients.

14. **T** **F** The Dental Assisting National Board (DANB) is the national certification for dental assistants.

15. **T** **F** The certified dental technician (CDT) must pass the Dental Assisting National Board (DANB) exam for certification.

Multiple Choice

1. Which of the following does the ADAA represent?

   a. hygienists

   b. assistants

   c. dentists

   d. laboratory technicians

2. Which of the following is not a member of the direct dental care team?

   a. dental hygienist

   b. dental laboratory technician

   c. dentist

   d. dental assistant

3. A dental laboratory technician is required to graduate from a CODA-accredited dental laboratory technician program. A laboratory technician seeking credentials must pass an examination administered by the National Board for Certification in Dental Laboratory Technology.

   a. Both statements are true.

   b. Both statements are false.

   c. The first statement is true; the second statement is false.

   d. The first statement is false; the second statement is true.

4. Which of the following is part of the direct dental care team?

   a. dental office manager

   b. dental assistant

   c. certified dental laboratory technician

   d. dental products salesperson

5. A dental hygienist who graduates from a 2- or 4-year program and obtains their RDH or LDH license is not able to perform which of the following as allowed by scope of practice?

   a. dental sealants

   b. extractions of teeth

   c. scaling

   d. root planing

CERTIFICATION REVIEW

1. Which of the following is correct about Dr. Greene Vardiman Black?

   a. He was an inventor of numerous machines for testing alloys.
   b. He was an inventor of numerous instruments to refine the cavity prep.
   c. He was known as the "grand old man of dentistry."
   d. All of the choices are correct.

2. Who first introduced infection control to England?

   a. Hesi-Re
   b. Alfred Fones
   c. Malvina Cueria
   d. Florence Nightingale

3. Who is recognized as the first dental assistant?

   a. Hesi-Re
   b. Alfred Fones
   c. Malvina Cueria
   d. Florence Nightingale

4. Who was the first dentist whose name was recorded in 3000 BC?

   a. Pierre Fauchard
   b. Hesi-Re
   c. John Greenwood
   d. Guy de Chauliac

5. Who was the first woman to graduate from a recognized dental college?

   a. Lucy Beaman Hobbs Taylor
   b. Ida Gray
   c. Juliette Southard
   d. Irene Morgan

6. Who helped to establish the first national association to represent the dental profession?

   a. James B. Morrison
   b. John Greenwood
   c. Josiah Flagg
   d. Chapin Harris

7. Who believed strongly that physicians should adhere to confidentiality?

   a. Florence Nightingale
   b. Hippocrates
   c. Josiah Flagg
   d. Juliette Southard

8. Who determined that dentists would not be able to be both surgeons and provide preventive treatments?

    a. Florence Nightingale

    b. Alfred C. Fones

    c. Chapen Harris

    d. Juliette Southard

9. Who formed the American Dental Hygienist Association?

    a. Florence Nightingale

    b. Alfred C. Fones

    c. Chapen Harris

    d. Juliette Southard

10. Who first advocated for disinfection of instruments with chemicals?

    a. Florence Nightingale

    b. Alfred C. Fones

    c. Joseph Lister

    d. Hesi-Re

CHAPTER APPLICATION

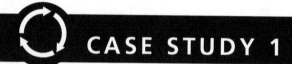

CASE STUDY 1

Gwen, age 18, is a first-year college student. She has occasionally experienced swollen gingiva behind her last molar. Now, it is final exam week and the swelling will not go down.

1. What should Gwen do?

    _____

    _____

    _____

2. What specialist would Gwen be referred to for resolving this condition?

    _____

    _____

    _____

CASE STUDY 2

Meridith, age 45, has recently been diagnosed with various oral conditions. A specialist is indicated to treat each of these conditions. What specialist will be sought for each of the following conditions?

1. Swollen gingiva and bone loss

_____

_____

2. Decay that has infected both the pulp canal and root/apex some of the front teeth

_____

_____

3. A third molar that needs to be extracted

_____

_____

4. An unknown soft tissue lesion

_____

_____

Critical Thinking

1. Name the four principles on which the American Dental Assistants Association was founded.

_____

_____

_____

2. There are certain benefits to membership in the American Dental Assistants Association.

    a. Name the benefits.

    _____

    _____

    _____

    b. What is the ADAA's website address?

    _____

    _____

3. Provide the year in which each of the following dentistry technologies was introduced or reported.

   a. Tooth morphology is identified _____ .

   b. Nitrous oxide is used for dental pain relief _____ .

   c. First commercially manufactured foot-treadle dental engine is patented _____ .

   d. First fluoride toothpastes are marketed _____ .

   e. Four-handed, sit-down dentistry is adopted _____ .

   f. First synthetic bristle (nylon) toothbrush is marketed _____ .

   g. Hepatitis B vaccine becomes available _____ .

   h. First reclining dental chair is invented _____ .

   i. Food and Drug Administration approves the use of the laser in removing tooth decay _____ .

   j. "Lost wax" casting machine is invented _____ .

   k. Osseointegration is introduced _____ .

   l. The x-ray is discovered _____ .

Psychology, Communication, and Multicultural Interaction

SPECIFIC INSTRUCTIONAL OBJECTIVES

The student should strive to meet the following objectives and demonstrate an understanding of the facts and principles presented in this chapter:

1. Use terms presented in this chapter.
2. Define psychology.
3. Compare and contrast the learning theories discussed in this chapter.
4. Discuss how Maslow's hierarchy of needs relates to communication in today's dental office.
5. Describe how defense mechanisms can inhibit communication.
6. Describe the components of the communication process.
7. Discuss dental phobias.
8. Define the factors that can affect communication.
9. Discuss how to achieve resolution in conflicts related to office stress.
10. Define cultural competency.
11. Compare and contrast culture, ethnicity, and race.
12. Discuss techniques to communicate with people from different cultures.
13. Identify the advantages and disadvantages of written communication.
14. Discuss ways to create effective written materials.
15. Discuss the steps involved in preparing for a dental presentation.
16. Design visuals that will enhance a presentation.
17. Develop strategies to communicate effectively during a presentation.

VOCABULARY BUILDER

Matching I

Match each term with the appropriate definition.

1. _____ auxiliary
2. _____ cognitive
3. _____ directive
4. _____ empathy
5. _____ encoding
6. _____ evidenced-based
7. _____ kinesthetic
8. _____ litigation
9. _____ nitrous oxide
10. _____ paradigm

a. gas that produces euphoria when inhaled
b. a person who provides additional support
c. widely accepted belief
d. mental process such as reasoning
e. information received through movement or lack of it
f. lawsuit
g. guidance
h. to convert a message
i. understand another's feelings
j. utilizing the findings of the current research

Matching II

Communication consists of five major process components. Match each term with its process.

Term

1. _____ sender
2. _____ message
3. _____ channel
4. _____ receiver
5. _____ feedback

Process

a. Communication medium in which message is sent
b. Formulated response, after decoding
c. Shapes the idea
d. Stimuli produced by the sender in written, verbal, or nonverbal form
e. Takes the message and makes sense of it

Fill in the Blank

Please fill in the blank with one of the choices provided.

Social Learning theory   Health Belief Model

Psychology   Stages of Change Theory

1. _____ is the science of the mind and of the reasons people think and act as they do.

2. The _____ views change as a process of stages over time rather than a single event.

3. The _____ is useful to predict whether a person will comply with your recommendations over a period of time.

4. The _____ is based on the theory that learning occurs in a series of sequential steps from being unaware of something to practicing a learned habit.

CHAPTER REVIEW

True or False

Circle whether the answer is true of false.

1. **T   F**   Abraham Maslow is considered the founder of a movement called *humanistic psychology*.

2. **T   F**   The dental assistant can communicate with and treat all patients in the same manner.

3. **T   F**   Encoding involves the use of specific signs, symbols, interpersonal communication, or language used in sending the message.

4. **T   F**   The kinesthetic channel of communication is hearing or listening to the verbal message.

5. **T   F**   Psychology is an acquired belief system that a person establishes through various life experiences.

6. **T   F**   Generation "Z" often rebels against the use of technology.

7. **T   F**   Patients with dental phobias have fear and severe anxiety that is excessive, unreasonable, and irrational, and they often are unable to overcome it without professional help.

8. **T   F**   One pharmacological technique used to treat patients with dental phobia is the use of nitrous oxide.

9. **T   F**   Stress is the body's method of reacting to specific conditions or a stimulus.

10. **T   F**   Office-related conflicts usually resolve themselves when they are ignored.

Multiple Choice

1. Using a caring touch demonstrates the use of which channel(s) to receive a message?

   a. auditory
   b. visual
   c. kinesthetic
   d. all of the above

2. Who or what begins the communication process?

   a. the message
   b. the sender
   c. the feedback
   d. the receiver

3. On average, how much time during the day do most college students spend talking?

   a. 15%
   b. 20%
   c. 25%
   d. 30%

4. What proportion of communication is verbal?

   a. 20%
   b. 40%
   c. 60%
   d. 80%

5. Which generation is often referred to as the "me generation"?

   a. Generation X
   b. Generation Y
   c. the MTV generation
   d. Baby Boomers

6. Which generation statistically holds the highest education levels?

    a. Generation X

    b. Generation Y

    c. Generation Y

    d. Baby Boomers.

7. Which generation is thought of as being highly connected?

    a. Generation X

    b. Generation Y

    c. Generation Z

    d. Baby Boomers

8. Within what distance does intimate touching usually occur?

    a. 3 inches

    b. 6 inches

    c. 9 inches

    d. 12 inches

9. If a patient is having difficulty breathing, which level of Maslow's hierarchy needs to be addressed?

    a. belongingness and love

    b. prestige and esteem

    c. self-actualization

    d. survival and physiological

10. Which of the following learning theories is also known as the decision-making continuum?

    a. Stages of Change Theory

    b. Maslow's hierarchy of needs

    c. Learning Ladder

    d. Health Belief Model

CERTIFICATION REVIEW

1. How can the dental team assist in providing optimal care to a patient?

    a. Scheduling the patient's appointment far into the future

    b. Ignoring the patient's complaints

    c. Being funny so the patient is entertained

    d. Encouraging the patient to ask questions and participate in treatment

2. What is an appropriate way to manage an anxious patient?

    a. Remain silent during patient appointments.

    b. Encourage questions during patient appointments.

    c. Move very slowly during the treatment appointments.

    d. Move very quickly during the treatment appointments.

3. Which of the following is the most important aspect of effective communication?

    a. good listening skills

    b. good nonverbal skills

    c. empathy skills

    d. good questioning skills

4. The patient that you will be assisting today is hearing impaired. What is the best way to communicate with this patient?

    a. Show pictures and speak softly.

    b. Speak slowly while maintaining eye contact.

    c. There is no need to speak as providing written materials is adequate.

    d. Draw pictures for the patient.

5. The patient who is in the patient chair is upset. What is the best way to manage this patient?

    a. Pay attention to what the patient is saying in a silent manner.
    b. Interrupt the patient so you can explain why the patient is wrong.
    c. Make comical statements so the patient starts to laugh.
    d. Leave the room and ignore the patient until she calms down.

6. You are assisting the dentist with a procedure and notice the patient is tightly gripping the arms of the chair with his hands. What form of communication is this?

    a. verbal
    b. nonverbal
    c. defense mechanism
    d. both verbal and nonverbal

7. The patient you are assisting with currently was born in 1993. What mode of communication regarding oral home care would be most effective with this patient?

    a. computer and the Internet
    b. printed pamphlets
    c. drawings with pen and paper
    d. strictly verbal communication

8. You seat the next patient in the treatment room, and the patient mentions she is anxious about the treatment. She has several questions that she would like to ask you. You realize that active listening is important. What is a characteristic of active listening?

    a. Setting up the operatory while the patient is asking her questions
    b. Texting your friend while the patient is asking her questions
    c. Giving the patient your undivided attention
    d. Ignoring what the patient says

9. Which of the following do not negatively affect patient–operator communication in the dental office?

    a. Making eye contact with the patient while they are speaking
    b. Staring out the window while the patient is speaking
    c. Cleaning up the operatory while the patient is speaking
    d. Answering a text message while the patient is speaking

10. You are working at the front desk of the dental office you are employed in. The phones are busy today, and several patients have called to make appointments. Which of the following is proper conduct regarding phone etiquette for effective communication?

    a. Speak in short sentences.
    b. Speak in a hard tone.
    c. The sitting position does not matter as the patient cannot see you.
    d. The facial expression effects the message to the caller.

CHAPTER APPLICATION

◯ CASE STUDY 1

Tyler presents to the office for an initial visit. Tyler is 43 years old and has poor oral health and has not been to a dentist for several years. He also has a diet high in sugar. The dental examination reveals multiple areas of decay. As you discuss his oral health care needs with him, he states, "My father had soft teeth, and I inherited them, which is why I have so many cavities."

1. What is Tyler using to explain why he has extensive decay?

   _____

   _____

   _____

2. Why might Tyler be using a defense mechanism?

   _____

   _____

   _____

3. What should the dental assistant do in this case?

   _____

   _____

   _____

✗ Critical Thinking

1. It is critical for a dental assistant to be a good listener and observer. During a dental procedure, the dental assistant notices that the patient is squeezing the dental chair arm and their knuckles are white.

   a. What is this method of communication?

   _____

   _____

   b. What can the dental assistant do in response to this communication to meet the patient's needs?

   _____

   _____

2. The dental assistant is speaking to a patient to explain proper flossing technique. While speaking to the patient, the dental assistant demonstrates the technique using a model of the teeth and some dental floss.

   a. What channel(s) of communication is the dental assistant using to send a message to the patient?

   _____

   _____

3. During a charting exercise, the dental assistant is uncertain about the tooth number, the surface, and the diagnosis to be charted.

   a. What communication skill is necessary for him or her to ensure a correct recording?

   _____

   _____

4. The dental assistant is speaking over the phone to a patient with a toothache who wishes to be seen as soon as possible.

   a. What actions can the dental assistant take to make sure the patient's needs are met and that the patient feels comfortable with how his or her needs are being addressed?

   _____

   _____

CHAPTER 3

Ethics, Jurisprudence, and the Health Information Portability and Accountability Act

SPECIFIC INSTRUCTIONAL OBJECTIVES

The student should strive to meet the following objectives and demonstrate an understanding of the facts and principles presented in this chapter:

1. Use terms presented in this chapter.

2. Define the ethical principles.

3. Determine approaches with possible outcomes to different ethical dilemmas.

4. Summarize the Professional Code of Conduct.

5. State what is covered by the Dental Practice Act.

6. Explain how jurisprudence is related to the dental assistant.

7. Discuss jurisprudence as it relates to civil law.

8. Discuss violations of the law in a dental setting.

9. Identify the agencies that influence dental practice.

10. Explain the individual roles of OSHA, EPA, FDA, CDC, OSAP, NIOSH.

11. Discuss HIPAA law.

12. Recall HIPAA practices in the dental office.

13. Relate HIPAA compliancy practices relative to third party requests.

14. Identify the responsibilities of the dental team in relation to HIPAA.

15. Explain under what conditions HIPAA information should be shared.

16. Recall HIPAA policies and practices in technology.

VOCABULARY BUILDER

Matching

Term	Definition
1. _____ ethical	a. false and malicious spoken words
2. _____ slander	b. do no harm
3. _____ informed consent	c. following principles of right and wrong
4. _____ beneficence	d. negligent professional activity or treatment
5. _____ autonomy	e. violation of trust
6. _____ breach	f. patient's agreement to care after being advised of benefits and risks
7. _____ jurisprudence	g. written law passed by legislative body
8. _____ malpractice	h. action done for the benefit of others
9. _____ statute	i. independence
10. _____ nonmaleficence	j. study of philosophy and law

Fill in the Blank

Please fill in the blank with one of the choices provided.

malpractice	privacy	Office of Civil Rights (OCR)
a contract	ethics	an expressed contract
defamation	expanded functions	
informed consent	doctrine of respondeat superior	

1. Like all functions that the auxiliary performs, the expanded functions fall under the
   _____ , which means "let the master answer."

2. Delegated functions that require increased responsibility and skill are called _____.

3. The _____ is the enforcement authority for transactions, code set identifiers, and
   security.

4. Each patient has the right to know and understand any procedure that is performed. The form that
   patients sign indicating they understand and accept treatment is called _____.

5. A contract that is written or verbal and that describes specifically what each party in the contract will do
   is called _____.

6. HIPAA requires that dental patients receive written notice of information practices, and an accounting of
   disclosures. The _____ official provides information to patients about their individual privacy
   rights and how their information may be used.

7. Defining what is right and wrong is called _____.

8. A binding agreement between two or more people is called _____.

9. A tort law protects against an individual causing injury to another person's reputation, name, or character.
   This injury is called _____.

10. The area of law covering any wrongful act that is a breach in due care that results in an injury to another person is called _____.

CHAPTER REVIEW

True or False

Circle whether the answer is true of false.

1. **T   F**   The office HIPAA manual must include a job description for each employee.

2. **T   F**   The office HIPPA manual must include disciplinary procedures for employees that violate HIPAA.

3. **T   F**   The risk of a security breach is high when using cell phone text messaging to discuss patient information.

4. **T   F**   It is acceptable to use one's own personal social media site to discuss patient cases without any patient identifiers.

5. **T   F**   Electronic health record systems must have passwords to prevent access to personal health information by unauthorized persons.

6. **T   F**   Omission or commission may result in a criminal lawsuit by a patient.

7. **T   F**   The employer is responsible for all functions of the dental assistant.

8. **T   F**   Nonregulatory agencies do not have the authority to mandate legal regulations.

Multiple Choice

1. Which is the area of law that governs dentistry?

   a. civil law
   b. criminal law
   c. dental jurisprudence
   d. common law

2. What is (are) enacted by each state legislative body to establish rules and regulations?

   a. State Board of Dentistry
   b. statutes
   c. Dental Practice Act
   d. reciprocity

3. What gives states the guidelines regarding eligibility for licensing and identifies the grounds by which this license can be suspended or repealed?

   a. dental jurisprudence
   b. Dental Practice Act
   c. State Board of Dentistry
   d. statutes

4. In some states, an individual who has passed the requirements for one state may apply for an agreement in another state to be allowed to perform dental skills without retaking a written or clinical exam. What is this called?

   a. contract
   b. consent
   c. reciprocity
   d. malpractice

5. What is the legal term used for the situation in which a dentist fails to notify a patient that he or she can no longer provide services?

   a. noncompliance
   b. due care
   c. negligence
   d. abandonment

6. The dentist and the dental team members have the responsibility and duty to perform due care in treating all patients. What is failure to do this is called?

    a. assault

    b. sufficient care

    c. malpractice

    d. abandonment

7. If a child refused treatment and the dental personnel threatened and restrained the child without parental consent, what charges could be brought?

    a. civil law

    b. criminal law

    c. assault and battery

    d. invasion of privacy

8. When a dentist sits down and the patient opens his or her mouth, what type of consent does this indicate?

    a. informed consent

    b. implied contract

    c. implied consent

    d. expressed contract

9. In the dental care setting, what is the most frequently exercised law?

    a. civil

    b. criminal

    c. common

    d. ethics

10. Which of the following are included in the American Dental Association's Principles of Ethics?

    1. justice
    2. veracity
    3. autonomy
    4. beneficence
    5. nonmaleficence
    6. education

    a. 1, 2, 3, 4, 6

    b. 2, 3, 4, 5, 6

    c. 1, 2, 3, 4, 5

    d. 1, 3, 4, 5, 6

11. In a dental office, patient records need to be protected. Which of the following is considered identifiable information and is protected by PHI rules?

    1. post-op instructions
    2. name
    3. aseptic techniques
    4. birth date
    5. telephone conversations
    6. telephone number

    a. 1, 2, 3

    b. 2, 4, 6

    c. 1, 3, 5

    d. 2, 3, 5

12. Which of the following may define personal ethics?

    1. family values
    2. personal experiences
    3. American Dental Association
    4. American Dental Assistants' Association
    5. culture
    6. society

    a. 1, 2, 5, 6

    b. 1, 2, 4, 6

    c. 1, 3, 5, 6

    d. 1, 2, 3, 5

CERTIFICATION REVIEW

1. A 17-year-old patient presents for treatment. Who should the consent for treatment be obtained from?

   a. legal guardian

   b. school principal

   c. dentist at the practice you are employed in

   d. the patient

2. In the event that a patient sues for malpractice, which form of consent would be beneficial to the dental practitioner?

   a. implied consent

   b. verbal consent

   c. inferred consent

   d. written consent

3. Why is it important for the dental assistant to be aware of their duties as outlined in each state's dental practice act?

   a. to be aware of which duties can be legally performed by the dental assistant

   b. to understand requirements related to OSHA

   c. to follow American Dental Association ethical guidelines

   d. to know the relevant HIPAA laws

4. The patient you are currently assisting the dentist with requires a referral to a specialist for further treatment. Which of the following is correct regarding the referral process?

   a. The patient will need to a sign a new informed consent prior to referral to a specialist.

   b. The patient will be required to sign a new HIPAA acknowledgement form prior to referral to a specialist.

   c. Advise the patient that since they will not be seen in the current office, the original records will be sent to the specialist.

   d. Advise the patient that a copy of their records will be sent to the specialist's office.

5. Which of the following is correct regarding OSHA?

   a. The purpose of OSHA is to protect the employer.

   b. The dentist is the only one required to comply with OSHA.

   c. All states are federally regulated by OSHA.

   d. All of the above are correct.

6. Dental assistants may be working in locations that are outside of the private practice such as correctional facilities and school settings. Select the correct statement below related to HIPAA information in public health areas of practice.

   a. A dental assistant working in a correctional facility does not need to follow HIPAA laws as the health information of inmates is excluded from HIPAA.

   b. The dental assistant should request that the correctional officer nearby leave in order to maintain privacy as this request may violate safety.

   c. The correctional facility should keep the health records of the inmate separate from the legal records of the inmate.

   d. It is never acceptable for a health care provider to share even minimal personal health information of the inmates with a correctional officer.

7. Select the correct response regarding HIPAA policies and practices related to technology.

    a. Online electronic transmission of personal health information must be protected under HIPAA.

    b. HIPAA does not mandate electronic storage of medical records; paper format is acceptable under HIPAA.

    c. Use of nonencrypted personal cell phones for personal health information transmission does not lead to HIPAA violations.

    d. Posting before and after treatment pictures of patients of the office is acceptable and does not violate HIPAA.

8. Which of the following is a not a violation of HIPAA following a team discussion about a patient?

    a. If the dental assistant is a friend of a patient in the office, it is allowable to share the patient's information with other people the patient may know.

    b. It is acceptable for the dental assistant to discuss personal information related to a patient during team discussions.

    c. The dental assistant must uphold HIPAA standards during team discussions.

    d. It is acceptable for the dental assistant to discuss a patient with a colleague so that patients in the waiting room can hear the conversation.

9. Which of the following is correct regarding the statute of limitation?

    a. The time limit for a patient to file a lawsuit is the same in all states in the United States.

    b. Generally, an injured patient may file a lawsuit within 5 years of the last date of treatment or within 3 years of the date that the injury was discovered.

    c. A patient can file a lawsuit at anytime after the injury was discovered and a statute of limitation does not apply.

    d. A statute of limitation is defined as the period of limitation for bringing forth certain types of legal action.

10. A wrongful act that results in injury to one person by another is a(n)

    a. tort.

    b. contract.

    c. assault.

    d. battery.

CHAPTER APPLICATION

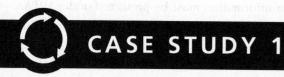

CASE STUDY 1

The receptionist in the dental office you are working in was recently hired. As you go to the reception area with the patient that was just completed, you hear the receptionist speaking with her friend, who is also a patient of the dental office. The receptionist is discussing another patient's medical history and mentions the patient's name.

1. What has the receptionist done wrong in this scenario?

_____

_____

_____

2. What should you do as the dental assistant?

_____

_____

_____

3. What legal action may take place in such a situation?

_____

_____

_____

X Critical Thinking

1. Explain the intent of the HIPAA Act of 1996.

_____

_____

_____

_____

_____

_____

2. You were recently hired as a dental assistant in a general practice office. You are at the front desk answering calls. You receive a call from someone who claims to be a social worker who is helping a patient of record of the office. The person requests the medical and dental records of the patient. What should be your next steps to ensure personal health information (PHI) is protected?

_____

_____

_____

_____

_____

_____

3. You are an assistant in a dental office. A patient presents to the office on an emergency basis due to pain in the lower right first molar. This patient has presented in the past for the same reason. In the past, the patient was provided with antibiotics and pain medication and was then scheduled to return for treatment of the tooth. The patient did not show up for the appointment. At this visit, the dentist provides a prescription for antibiotics and pain medication. You explain to the patient that they must return to complete treatment. The patient is scheduled for the following week. The patient again does not show up for treatment. Can the patient be dismissed from the office as a patient of record?

_____

_____

_____

_____

_____

_____

Dental Sciences

CHAPTER 4

General Anatomy and Physiology

SPECIFIC INSTRUCTIONAL OBJECTIVES

The student should strive to meet the following objectives and demonstrate an understanding of the facts and principles presented in this chapter:

1. Use terms presented in this chapter.

2. List the body systems, body planes and directions, and cavities of the body, and describe the structure and function of the cell.

3. Explain the functions and divisions of the skeletal system, list the composition of the bone, and identify the types of joints.

4. List the functions and structure of the muscular system.

5. List the functions and structure of the nervous system.

6. List the functions and structure of the endocrine system.

7. Explain dental concerns related to the reproductive system.

8. List the functions and structure of the circulatory system.

9. List the functions and structure of the digestive system.

10. List the functions and structure of the respiratory system.

11. List the functions and structure of the lymphatic system and the immune system.

12. List the functions and structure of the integumentary system.

13. List the functions and structure of the urinary system.

VOCABULARY BUILDER

Matching I

Match each term with the appropriate definition.

1. _____ epidermis

2. _____ epinephrine

3. _____ erythrocyte

4. _____ epithelial

a. lines body structures

b. hormone helps body meet physical stress

c. red blood cell transporting oxygen to tissue

d. outer layer of the skin

Matching II

Match each term with the appropriate definition.

1. _____ epi-

2. _____ erythro-

3. _____ leuko-

4. _____ oss, osteo

5. _____ autonomic

6. _____ articulation

7. _____ coagulation

8. _____ homeostasis

9. _____ lymph

10. _____ macrophage

11. _____ periosteum

12. _____ sphincter

a. red

b. bone

c. on upon

d. white

e. process of forming a clot

f. involuntary, unconscious functions

g. connection of movable parts

h. maintaining a stable environment

i. engulfs and ingests infectious microorganism

j. membrane that covers the surface of bones

k. circular muscle constricting an opening

l. fluid that removes bacteria from tissue

Fill in the Blank

Please fill in the blank with one of the choices provided.

tendon	cancellous	glucose
ligament	mucous	bones
cortical	mucus	muscle

1. The major source of energy for the body is _____.

2. The _____ bone is the dense, outer layer of bone. The porous bone structure is _____ bone.

3. The _____ membranes line the body cavities and secrete _____ to lubricate and protect the lining.

4. The _____ is the attachment of muscle to bones. The connective tissue connecting the ends of the bones is the _____.

CHAPTER REVIEW

True or False

1. Arteries carry oxygenated blood from the heart to the body. Veins carry deoxygenated blood from the body back to the heart.

    a. Both statements are true.
    b. Both statements are false.
    c. The first statement is true; the second statement is false.
    d. The first statement is false; the second statement is true.

2. The esophagus is the passage for air to and from the lungs. The trachea is the passage connecting the throat to the stomach.

    a. Both statements are true.
    b. Both statements are false.
    c. The first statement is true; the second statement is false.
    d. The first statement is false; the second statement is true.

3. The sagittal plane divides the body into upper and lower sections. The frontal plane divides the body into the left and right halves.

    a. Both statements are true.
    b. Both statements are false.
    c. The first statement is true; the second statement is false.
    d. The first statement is false; the second statement is true.

Multiple Choice

1. Which component of the cell is made up mostly of water and suspends other cell structures?

    a. cell membrane
    b. cytoplasm
    c. microvilli
    d. lipid

2. Which tissue lines the body structures?

    a. epithelial
    b. muscular
    c. connective
    d. nervous

3. Which describes a structure near the surface of the body?

    a. medial
    b. superior
    c. anterior
    d. superficial

4. In what part of the bone are blood cells?

    a. cancellous
    b. cortical
    c. periosteum
    d. marrow

5. Which is lined by fluid and is free moving?

    a. cartilaginous
    b. fibrous
    c. synovial
    d. fibrous and synovial

6. What are the functions of the skeletal system?

    a. to provide framework, support the body, and protect organs

    b. support, heat production, and movement

    c. communication throughout the body

    d. to produce and secrete hormones to maintain a healthy, functioning body

7. What is the function of the muscular system?

    a. to provide framework, support the body, and protect organs

    b. support of the body, heat production, and movement

    c. communication throughout the body

    d. to produce and secrete hormones to maintain a healthy, functioning body

8. What is the function of the nervous system?

    a. to provide framework, support of the body and protection of organs

    b. support the body, heat production and movement healthy, functioning body

    c. communication throughout the body by electrical impulses

    d. produce and secrete hormones to maintain

9. Which is the largest section of the brain and controls thoughts, memory, and language?

    a. cerebrum

    b. cerebellum

    c. brain stem

    d. diencephalon

10. What is the function of the endocrine system?

    a. to provide framework, support the body, and protect organs

    b. support the body, heat production, and movement

    c. communication throughout the body by electrical impulses

    d. produce and secrete hormones to maintain healthy, functioning body

11. Which is located below the urinary bladder, surrounds the urethra, and if enlarged may cause difficulty with urination?

    a. urinary meatus

    b. prostate

    c. vas deferens

    d. epididymis

12. Which is a sac-like structure that cushions the heart and reduces friction of the beating heart?

    a. endocardium

    b. myocardium

    c. epicardium

    d. apex

13. The _____ acts like the pacemaker causing the heart's electrical impulse to begin.

    a. atrioventricular node

    b. sinoatrial node

    c. bundle of His

    d. Purkinje fibers

14. Which helps protect the body from harmful pathogens and foreign materials?

    a. erythrocytes

    b. leukocytes

    c. thrombocytes

    d. Rh factor

15. What is the function of the digestive system?

    a. bring fresh air into lungs, allow gas exchange, and remove waste
    b. support the body, heat production, and movement
    c. break down food, absorb nutrients, and eliminate solid waste
    d. produce and secrete hormones to maintain healthy, functioning body

16. Where does the major absorption of nutrients from food occur?

    a. oral cavity
    b. esophagus
    c. small intestine
    d. large intestine

17. Which is one of the largest organs that processes nutrients and detoxifies harmful substances?

    a. liver
    b. gallbladder
    c. pancreas
    d. salivary gland

18. What is the function of the diaphragm?

    a. separates the stomach and lungs
    b. pushes air out of the lungs
    c. contracts for inhalation
    d. raises the rib cage

19. What regulates the respiration rate?

    a. oxygen levels in the blood
    b. carbon dioxide levels in the blood
    c. size of the patient
    d. age of the patient

20. Which is very vascular, filters the blood, destroys old red blood cells and pathogens, and stores blood?

    a. thymus
    b. lymph nodes
    c. bladder
    d. spleen

21. Where do the lymph vessels carry extra fluid from the tissue after it is filtered?

    a. digestive system
    b. respiratory system
    c. urinary system
    d. circulatory system

22. Which layer of skin has a rich blood supply and contains all the accessory organs?

    a. dermis
    b. epidermis
    c. subcutaneous
    d. keratin

23. Which integumentary accessory glands helps maintain the body temperature throughout the body?

    a. sebaceous
    b. sweat
    c. apocrine
    d. melanin

24. Which organ could be nicknamed the filtering station?

    a. ureter
    b. bladder
    c. urethra
    d. kidney

25. How many bones are in the adult skeleton?

    a. 300
    b. 200
    c. 216
    d. 206

26. If muscles are not used, they begin to deteriorate. What is this condition known as?

    a. atrophy
    b. fibromyalgia
    c. spasticity
    d. gravis

27. What are the nerve fibers that conduct impulses to the cell body?

a. axons

b. dendrites

c. synapses

d. myelin

CERTIFICATION REVIEW

Multiple Choice

1. The basic atomic structure consists of _____.

   1. atoms

   2. neutrons

   3. protons

   4. electrons

     a. 1, 2

     b. 1, 3

     c. 2, 3, 4

     d. 1, 3, 4

2. Which statement describes molecules?

   a. the smallest component of an element

   b. combination of two or more atoms

   c. come together to form tissues

   d. form organs

3. Which is also referred to as spongy bone?

   a. cortical

   b. cancellous

   c. compound

   d. trabeculae

4. What is the muscle origin?

   a. beginning of where the muscles attach

   b. where the muscle ends

   c. attachment to more movable bone

   d. attachment to ligament

5. Which statement describes the trachea?

   a. also referred to as voice box

   b. tubes that enter the lungs

   c. also referred to as windpipe

   d. where exchange of oxygen and carbon dioxide occurs

6. What is the membrane that divides a cavity into two parts?

    a. septum
    b. chamber
    c. capillary
    d. frenum

7. The pituitary gland is part of what body system?

    a. endocrine
    b. nervous
    c. integumentary
    d. cardiovascular

8. What is the thin lining on the inside of the heart?

    a. pericardium
    b. myocardium
    c. endocardium
    d. atrium

9. Which statement describes isotonic movement?

    a. Muscles stretch or spread in order to perform tasks.
    b. Tension in the muscular system decreases.
    c. Length of muscle is not changed, but tension increases.
    d. Muscle tension remains the same but muscles shorten.

10. Which transmits genetic information, is in the nucleus, and contains DNA?

    a. cell membrane
    b. chromosome
    c. ribosome
    d. cytoplasm

CHAPTER APPLICATION

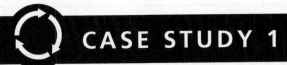 **CASE STUDY 1**

A scheduled dental appointment has brought Yuri in today for a filling. Before treatment, in response to a query by the dental assistant about changes in her health history since the last appointment, Yuri said that she is pregnant.

1. Which body system is most affected by pregnancy?

_____

_____

_____

2. How do changes in hormones and diet during pregnancy affect the mother's oral health? How can this affect the developing baby?

_____

_____

_____

_____

_____

3. What, if any, dental treatment might be affected during pregnancy?

_____

_____

_____

_____

Critical Thinking

1. When a patient has low bone density, what would be charted in the medical records?

_____

_____

Questions 2 and 3: Tuberculosis is documented on the patient's medical history form. The dental assistant needs to be knowledgeable about this disease.

2. What body system is affected?

_____

_____

3. How can it be transmitted to the assistant?

_____

_____

_____

Image Labeling

Label the following basic cell structures.

cell membrane

chromosomes

cytoplasm

nucleus

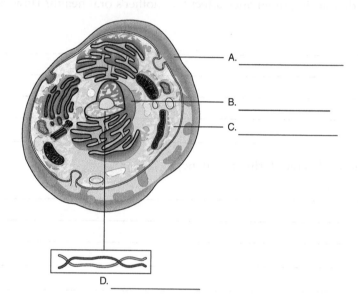

A. _____

B. _____

C. _____

D. _____

CHAPTER 5

Head and Neck Anatomy

SPECIFIC INSTRUCTIONAL OBJECTIVES

The student should strive to meet the following objectives and demonstrate an understanding of the facts and principles presented in this chapter:

1. Use terms presented in this chapter.

2. Identify the bones of the cranium.

3. Identify the landmarks of the face and the oral cavity, including the tongue, floor of the mouth, and salivary glands.

4. Label the landmarks that are important in dentistry of the following: maxilla, mandible, and sphenoid bone.

5. Describe how the parts of the TMJ are involved in the articulation and movement of the joint.

6. Discuss the possible problems associated with the TMJ.

7. Discuss the functions of the following: muscles of the head, muscles of mastication, muscles of facial expression, the floor of the mouth, the tongue, muscles of the neck.

8. Describe the structure of the tongue.

9. Discuss the salivary glands.

10. Discuss the salivary secretions.

11. Describe the major divisions of the nervous system.

12. Identify the nerves of the maxilla and the mandible.

13. List the areas innervated by each cranial nerve in order by name and Roman numeral.

14. Explain in detail the innervation of the major divisions of the trigeminal nerve.

15. Discuss the pathway of blood in the body.

16. Discuss in detail, the arteries and veins of the head, neck, tongue, teeth, and face.

17. Discuss the location of the important lymph nodes in dentistry.

18. Explain why a patient head and neck exam is important during a dental visit.

VOCABULARY BUILDER

Matching I

Match the following terms with the correct definition.

1. _____ afferent
2. _____ amylase
3. _____ anguli
4. _____ antigen
5. _____ canthus
6. _____ dorsum
7. _____ efferent
8. _____ eminence
9. _____ fissure
10. _____ foramen
11. _____ fossa
12. _____ innervate
13. _____ labii
14. _____ lacuna
15. _____ maxillary
16. _____ palatine
17. _____ palpate
18. _____ trismus
19. _____ ventral
20. _____ xerostomia

a. enzyme in saliva that starts the digestion process
b. corner of the mouth
c. substance foreign to the body
d. corner of the eye
e. carrying information to a central organ
f. upper, outer surface of an organ
g. projection of bone
h. groove or natural division
i. passage or opening
j. carries motor impulses away from central organ
k. pertaining to lips
l. shallow depression
m. to supply a body part with nerves
n. pertaining to upper arch of the oral cavity
o. tiny cavity in substance of bone
p. underside of tongue
q. lockjaw
r. to examine by touch
s. related to roof of the oral cavity
t. dry mouth

CHAPTER REVIEW

Multiple Choice

1. Which is the largest salivary gland?

   a. parotid
   b. submandibular

   c. sublingual caruncles
   d. sublingual

2. From which gland does the Wharton's duct empty saliva?

   a. parotid
   b. fauces

   c. submandibular
   d. terminalis

3. Which bone contains the mastoid process?

   a. parietal
   b. temporal

   c. frontal
   d. occipital

4. Which bone is a single continuous bone that goes across the anterior of the skull to the temporal bones and is shaped like a bat with its wings spread?

   a. styloid
   b. occipital

   c. sphenoid
   d. pterygoid

5. Which bone forms the cheeks?

   a. vomer
   b. nasal

   c. lacrimal
   d. zygomatic

6. The tear ducts pass through which bones?

   a. zygomatic
   b. nasal

   c. vomer
   d. lacrimal

7. Which of the following bones has two sections and is the largest of the facial bones?

   a. maxilla
   b. mandible

   c. palatine
   d. rami

8. Which of the following is the only movable bone of the face?

   a. maxilla
   b. mandible

   c. rami
   d. palatine

9. What is the function of the temporal muscles of mastication?

   a. depress the mandible
   b. depress the maxilla

   c. expand the posterior fibers
   d. elevate the mandible

10. The masseter muscles belong to which group of muscles of the head and neck?

    a. muscles of facial expression
    b. muscles of the floor of the mouth

    c. muscles of the tongue
    d. muscles of mastication

11. The buccinator muscle group belongs to which of the following?

    a. muscles of facial expression
    b. muscles of the floor of the mouth

    c. muscles of the tongue
    d. muscles of mastication

12. Which of the following muscles functions to wrinkle the skin of the chin?

    a. buccinator
    b. masseter
    c. orbicularis oris
    d. mentalis

13. Which of the following muscles serves to form the floor of the mouth?

    a. digastric
    b. genioglossus
    c. hypoglossus
    d. styloglossus

14. Which of the following cranial nerves is the largest and innervates the maxilla and the mandible?

    a. ophthalmic
    b. trigeminal
    c. nasopalatine
    d. infraorbital

15. Which nerve branch is composed of both sensory and motor fibers?

    a. lingual
    b. inferior alveolar
    c. buccal
    d. optic

16. The buccal nerve branch innervates which of the following?

    1. lingual mucosa
    2. buccal mucosa
    3. buccal gingiva of the mandibular molars
        a. 1, 3
        b. 1, 2, 3
        c. 2, 3

17. Which of the following is not correct regarding the external jugular vein?

    a. receives blood from the external part of the cranium
    b. receives blood from the deeper structures of the face
    c. drains directly into the right atrium of the heart
    d. drains blood from the structures around the maxilla and the mandible

18. Which of the following is not correct regarding the internal jugular vein?

    a. receives blood from the brain
    b. drains blood from pterygoid plexus
    c. drains blood from the maxillary vein
    d. drains directly into the right atrium of the heart

19. The largest papillae, which are mushroom shaped, are anterior to the sulcus terminalis in a row of 8 to 10. What are these called?

    a. filiform papillae
    b. fungiform papillae
    c. foliate papillae
    d. circumvallate papillae

20. What of the following articulates with the temporal bones to form the temporomandibular joint?

    a. palatine
    b. condyle
    c. foramen
    d. symphysis

Matching II

Match each minor salivary gland with the correct location provided.

1. _____ labial
2. _____ buccal
3. _____ palatine
4. _____ glossopalatini
5. _____ anterior lingual
6. _____ von Ebner's

a. soft palate and posterior 2/3 hard palate
b. near tip of tongue
c. lips
d. inner cheek
e. posterior lateral palate
f. dorsum of base of tongue

Matching III

Match each cranial nerve with the correct description.

1. _____ trigeminal
2. _____ facial
3. _____ olfactory
4. _____ optic

a. innervates muscles of facial expression
b. functions in the sense of smell
c. functions in the sense of sight
d. multiple functions in head and oral cavity

CERTIFICATION REVIEW

1. How many bones make up the cranium?

   a. 16
   b. 12
   c. 10
   d. 22

2. Which duct drains the sublingual salivary glands?

   a. Wharton's duct
   b. ducts of Rivinus
   c. Stensen's duct
   d. duct of Bartholin

3. Which duct drains the sublingual salivary glands?

   a. Wharton's duct
   b. ducts of Rivinus
   c. Stensen's duct
   d. duct of Bartholin

4. Which of the following bones of the neurocranium is a paired bone?

   a. occipital

   b. frontal

   c. temporal

   d. sphenoid

5. Which of the following mandibular structures is the entrance to the inferior alveolar canal?

   a. lingula

   b. mandibular foramen

   c. mental foramen

   d. coronoid process

6. Which of the following is the largest of the muscles of mastication?

   a. temporalis

   b. masseter

   c. internal pteryogoid

   d. external pterygoid

7. Which of the following is the strongest of the muscles of mastication?

   a. temporalis

   b. masseter

   c. internal pterygoid

   d. external pterygoid

8. Which of the following muscles of the neck originates in the occipital bone and inserts in the clavicle and shoulder bone?

   a. masseter

   b. sternocleidomastoid

   c. trapezius

   d. platysma

9. Which of the following structures of the tongue is the embryonic origin of the thyroid gland?

   a. foramen cecum

   b. sulcus terminalis

   c. lingual foramen

   d. median lingual sulcus

10. Which of the following salivary glands produce approximately 1/5 of the total saliva produced?

   a. sublingual

   b. submandibular

   c. parotid

   d. labial

CHAPTER APPLICATION

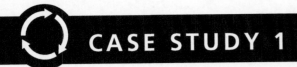

CASE STUDY 1

Sara, a patient of record, is being prepared for dental treatment. The dental assistant asks Sara if there has been any change in her health since her last appointment. Sara states that her mouth "is extremely dry lately."

1. What is the function of saliva?

_____

_____

_____

2. What are the three major salivary glands and their functions?

_____

_____

_____

_____

_____

_____

_____

_____

3. How much saliva should a person produce each day?

_____

_____

4. What may cause xerostomia?

_____

_____

 Critical Thinking

Palpation of the head and neck lymph nodes should be a common practice during an extra-oral examination.

1. Which lymph node areas important in dentistry should be palpated?

2. Why is this an important part of the dental exam?

_____

_____

_____

_____

_____

_____

The trigeminal nerve is an important nerve in dentistry.

3. What are the three divisions of the trigeminal nerve?

_____

_____

_____

4. Which branch(es) of the trigeminal nerve is/are purely sensory?

_____

_____

_____

5. What are the two types of movement of the TMJ?

_____

_____

6. What are the types of problems that can occur with the TMJ?

_____

_____

_____

CHAPTER 6

Landmarks of the Face and Oral Cavity

SPECIFIC INSTRUCTIONAL OBJECTIVES

The student should strive to meet the following objectives and demonstrate an understanding of the facts and principles presented in this chapter:

1. Use terms presented in this chapter.
2. Identify landmarks in each region of the face.
3. Identify landmarks in the oral cavity.
4. Discuss the boundaries of each division of the oral cavity.
5. List the structures in each division of the oral cavity.
6. Discuss the soft tissues that surround the dentition.

VOCABULARY BUILDER

Matching

Match each term with the appropriate definition.

1. _____ ala
2. _____ exostosis
3. _____ fauces
4. _____ frenulum
5. _____ midpalatal raphe
6. _____ palatal torus
7. _____ philtrum
8. _____ retromolar pad
9. _____ vermillion border
10. _____ vestibule

a. ridge of oral mucosa that marks median of hard palate

b. fold of mucous membrane that attaches two areas

c. indentation on upper lip below the tip of the nose

d. formation of bony growth

e. area between oral cavity and soft palate

f. tissue on mandibular alveolar process behind last molar

g. bony growth on roof of oral cavity

h. space between cheeks and teeth

i. flared portion of outside of nostril

j. line of color change between lip margin and skin

Fill in the Blank

Please fill in the blank with one of the choices provided.

adenoid	attached gingiva	fovea palatine
labiomental groove	Fordyce granules	posterior nasal spine
linea alba	mucogingival junction	
maxillary tuberosity	palatal rugae	

1. The sharp, pointed medial end of posterior border of the union of the palatal bones is the _____.

2. The depression that passes between the lower lip and the chin is known as the _____.

3. The ridges of mucosa that are present on the anterior portion of the roof of the oral cavity are known as _____.

4. The junction of the free mucosa of the cheeks and floor of the oral cavity and the gingiva is known as the _____.

5. The intraoral soft tissue that is firmly bound to the tooth and alveolar process is known as the _____.

6. The two small depressions found on or near the junction of the soft palate to hard palate are known as _____.

7. Sebaceous glands, which are visible on the inner surface of the cheek and the vermilion border, are known as _____.

8. The bulge posterior to the last maxillary molar is known as _____.

9. The white horizontal line which is level with the biting plane and on the mucosal surface of the cheek is known as _____.

10. Lymphoid tissue which is found in the upper pharynx is known as _____.

CHAPTER REVIEW

True or False

Circle whether the answer is true of false.

1. **T   F**   The area on the face around the eyes is known as the frontal region.

2. **T   F**   The area of the face which includes the forehead is known as the infraorbital region.

3. **T   F**   Line alba can be found unilaterally or bilaterally.

4. **T   F**   Extra bone that develops on the buccal surface of the maxilla or the mandible is known as an exostosis.

5. **T   F**   The corners of the mouth where the upper lip meets the lower lip are known as the labial commissures.

6. **T   F**   The top surface of the tongue is called the dorsal surface.

7. **T   F**   The smallest papilla on the dorsal surface of the tongue are known as circumvallate papilla.

8. **T   F**   The lingual frenum attaches the dorsal surface of the tongue to the floor of the mouth.

9. **T   F**   Enamel, which covers the crowns of the teeth, is the strongest tissue in the body.

10. **T   F**   The roots of the teeth are covered in cementum.

Multiple Choice

1. What is the area of the forehead between and above the eyebrows called?

   a. glabella
   b. ala

   c. commissure
   d. sulcus

2. What is the outer edge of the nostril called?

   a. ala of the nose
   b. philtrum

   c. commissure
   d. sulcus

3. What forms the inferior and superior margins of the oral vestibule?

   a. vestibular fornix
   b. philtrum

   c. vermilion border
   d. commissures

4. What is the soft tissue that lines the inner surface of the lips and cheeks called?

   a. papilla
   b. gingiva

   c. frenum
   d. mucosa

5. What is the name of the junction of the body of the mandible with the ramus of the mandible?

   a. angle of the mandible
   b. zygomatic arch

   c. frontal region
   d. mandibular tori

6. What is the name of the raised bump of tissue behind the maxillary central incisors?

   a. palatal rugae
   b. midpalatine raphe

   c. maxillary tuberosity
   d. incisive papilla

7. What is the roof of the oral cavity called?

   a. frenum
   b. palate

   c. tonsils
   d. papilla

8. What is the name of the structure that hangs down from the soft palate into the fauces and aids in swallowing?

   a. uvula
   b. tonsil

   c. adenoids
   d. papilla

9. Which papilla are the most numerous on the dorsal surface of the tongue and give the tongue its velvety texture?

   a. circumvallate papillae
   b. filiform papillae

   c. fungiform papillae
   d. foliate papillae

10. What is the name of area the soft tissue area that is located on either side of the lingual frenum?

   a. sublingual caruncles
   b. sublingual folds

   c. sublingual gland
   d. sebaceous gland

CERTIFICATION REVIEW

1. What portion of the tooth is covered with enamel?

   a. anatomical crown

   b. clinical crown

   c. root

   d. pulp

2. What substance covers the root of the tooth?

   a. enamel

   b. dentin

   c. cementum

   d. periodontal ligament

3. What tooth tissues join at the cervix of the tooth?

   a. cementum and pulp

   b. enamel and pulp

   c. enamel and dentin

   d. enamel and cementum

4. Which of the following is correct about dentin?

   a. It makes up the bulk of the tooth.

   b. It is under the enamel of the tooth crown.

   c. It is present in the root of the tooth.

   d. Is covered by cementum in the root of the tooth.

      i. a, b, c, d

     ii. a, b, c

    iii. a, b, d

    iv. b, c, d

5. When the lips are pulled out, raised lines of mucosal tissue extend from the alveolar mucosa through the vestibule to the labial and buccal mucosa. What are these are called?

   a. incisive papilla

   b. frena

   c. buccal mucosa

   d. parotid papilla

6. The largest papillae, which are mushroom shaped, are anterior to the sulcus terminalis in a row of 8 to 10. What are these called?

   a. filiform papillae

   b. fungiform papillae

   c. foliate papillae

   d. circumvallate papillae

7. The teeth are embedded in which structure of the oral cavity?

    a. cementum

    b. dentin

    c. enamel

    d. alveolar bone

8. Healthy gingival tissues are usually coral pink. However, many people have some pigmentation present in the tissues. What is this pigmentation called?

    a. enamel

    b. dentin

    c. melanin

    d. mucosa

9. What is the name of the triangular soft tissue between adjacent teeth?

    a. interdental papilla

    b. mucosa

    c. epithelial attachment

    d. free gingiva

10. Which of the following is correct regarding the mucogingival junction (MGJ)?

    a. It is more keratinized than the tissue that lines the inside of the cheeks.

    b. It is the junction between the attached gingiva and alveolar mucosa.

    c. The mucogingival junction is a straight line.

    d. All of the choices are correct.

CHAPTER APPLICATION

 CASE STUDY 1

A long-time patient of the dental office calls and is very upset. She states that she would like to be seen immediately as she has noticed a growth on the roof of her mouth. She is concerned that it may be cancer. The patient is scheduled for later that afternoon. You seat her in the operatory and review her medical history. The patient is extremely worried and tells you about the recently discovered growth on the roof of her mouth. While waiting for the dentist to come in you take a look and realize it is a small bony lump on the center of her palate.

1. What do you think this bump is?

    _____

    _____

2. What do you explain to the patient?

    _____

    _____

CASE STUDY 2

A new patient presents for an exam. When the patient is asked to lift her tongue, she is only able to do so in a limited manner.

1. What might be causing this limited movement?

   _____

   _____

2. What is the term for this problem?

   _____

   _____

Critical Thinking

1. What are the boundaries of the oral cavity?

   _____

   _____

   _____

2. Due to infection, the palatine tonsils are often marked with deep grooves and are red and inflamed. Describe their location.

   _____

   _____

   _____

   _____

3. Describe the function of the palatine tonsils.

   _____

   _____

   _____

4. The area of the oral cavity, which is sometimes under the tongue on the alveolar bone, sometimes has excess bone formation. What is this excess bone formation called?

   _____

   _____

   _____

5. You are assisting the dental hygienist with a patient cleaning. The dental hygienist completed the oral exam and dries the tissues while examining the soft tissues. You note that the tissue is healthy and has an "orange peel appearance." What is this appearance called?

_____

_____

_____

6. The dental hygienist now begins to probe, and you are recording probing depths. Where does the dental hygienist insert the periodontal probe to obtain the probing depths?

_____

_____

_____

Embryology and Histology

SPECIFIC INSTRUCTIONAL OBJECTIVES

The student should strive to meet the following objectives and demonstrate an understanding of the facts and principles presented in this chapter:

1. Use terms presented in this chapter.
2. Discuss the developmental stages of the human from fertilization to birth.
3. Describe the development of the human face.
4. Discuss the development of the following structures of the oral cavity: upper lip, palate, and tongue.
5. Discuss the role of the pharyngeal arches in the development of the structures of the face.
6. Identify the mechanism leading to development of a cleft palate.
7. Describe the various stages of tooth development.
8. Describe the function of the following in relation to tooth development: dental papilla, dental sacs, and enamel organ.
9. Describe changes that occur in the inner enamel epithelial cells as they mature to become ameloblasts.
10. Describe the structural properties of enamel.
11. Describe the structural properties of dentin.
12. Differentiate among the various types of dentin.
13. Discuss the formation of cementum.
14. Define artifacts that may occur in enamel, dentin, or cementum.
15. Describe each of the four tissues of a tooth.
16. State the components of the periodontium.
17. Describe the structure of the following: alveolar process, cementum, periodontal ligament, and gingiva.
18. Define the junctions of the tissues.

VOCABULARY BUILDER

Matching

Match each term with the appropriate definition.

1. _____ alveolar crest	a. directed toward the head
2. _____ ameloblast	b. residual cells from Hertwig's epithelial root sheath
3. _____ apposition	c. middle layer of the three primary germ layers
4. _____ caudal	d. primitive oral cavity
5. _____ cephalic	e. fertilized egg
6. _____ dentinal tubule	f. highest point of alveolar bone between teeth
7. _____ ectoderm	g. pertaining to posterior of body
8. _____ enamel organ	h. innermost of the three primary germ layers
9. _____ endoderm	i. to insert one part of a structure within a part of the same structure
10. _____ epithelial rests of Malassez	j. membrane which divides nasal cavity in half
11. _____ Hertwig's epithelial root sheath	k. layer of enamel organ between IEE and stellate reticulum
12. _____ inorganic	l. cells that form enamel
13. _____ invagination	m. tubes within dentin
14. _____ mesoderm	n. bulk of enamel organ
15. _____ nasal septum	o. outer layer of cells in an embryo
16. _____ olfactory pits	p. deposition of successive layers of material
17. _____ stellate reticulum	q. also known as nasal pits
18. _____ stomodeum	r. cells that guide shape of root during development
19. _____ stratum intermedium	s. not formed by a living organism
20. _____ zygote	t. part of tooth germ that forms enamel of tooth

CHAPTER REVIEW

Multiple Choice

1. In which week of prenatal development will the face begin to form?

   a. twelfth
   b. fourth
   c. sixteenth
   d. ninth

2. In the facial development phase, which embryonic layer is responsible for forming the upper portion of the face, forehead, eyes, and bridge of nose?

   a. median nasal
   b. mandibular process
   c. frontonasal process
   d. stomodeum

3. In the facial development phase, which embryonic layer is responsible for forming the cheeks, sides of the upper lip, and maxilla?

   a. median nasal process
   b. mandibular process
   c. frontonasal process
   d. stomodeum

4. Which factors can initiate malformation in the unborn child?

   a. genetics

   b. environment

   c. infections

   d. all of the above

5. What is it called when a cleft lip occurs on both sides of the lip?

   a. unilateral

   b. bilateral

   c. complete

   d. partial

6. What is the first stage of the life cycle of the tooth is called?

   a. initiation

   b. lamina

   c. odontogenesis

   d. proliferation

7. Enamel-forming cells are called

   a. odontoblasts.

   b. cementoblasts.

   c. ameloblasts.

   d. buds.

8. What is the last stage of tooth development before eruption?

   a. apposition

   b. bud

   c. cap

   d. bell

9. Which cells form the bones of the mandible and the maxilla?

   a. osteoblasts

   b. osteoclasts

   c. alveolus

   d. lamina

10. Which are the cells that remodel and resorb bone?

    a. osteoblasts

    b. osteoclasts

    c. alveolus

    d. lamina

11. What is the area where the buccal and lingual cortical bone plates come together between each tooth called?

    a. alveolar crest

    b. alveolus

    c. alveolar process

    d. lamina dura

12. What is the name of the radiopaque line seen on the dental radiograph that represents the lining of the bony tooth socket?

    a. alveolar crest

    b. periodontal ligament

    c. alveolar process

    d. lamina dura

Matching

Match the following terms with their correct definitions.

1. _____ enamel lamella

2. _____ enamel tuft

3. _____ enamel spindle

   a. short, dentinal tubules that may have crossed over into the enamel and were trapped there during the process of enamel mineralization

b. short hypocalcified structures that extend from the dentinoenamel junction and extend slightly into the enamel

c. narrower and longer hypocalcified structures that extend from the dentinoenamel junction and into the enamel

Match each tissue junction with the correct definition.

1. _____ dentinoenamel junction (DEJ)

2. _____ cementoenamel junction (CEJ)

3. _____ dentocemental junction (CDJ)

   a. where the dentin meets the cementum

   b. where the dentin meets the enamel

   c. where the cementum meets the enamel

CERTIFICATION REVIEW

1. Which of the following embryonic layers differentiates into enamel and the lining of the oral cavity?

   a. ectoderm

   b. mesoderm

   c. endoderm

   d. stomodeum

2. Which of the following processes forms the olfactory pits?

   a. lateral nasal

   b. frontal

   c. median nasal

   d. globular

3. Which of the following layers of the bell stage is responsible for nourishing the developing ameloblasts?

   a. outer enamel epithelium

   b. inner enamel epithelium

   c. stellate reticulum

   d. stratum intermedium

4. Which of the following is not correct regarding the structure of enamel?

   a. Enamel is laid down in increments, which results in striae of Retzius.

   b. Hydroxyapatite crystals are deposited into amelogenin, causing mineralization.

   c. The enamel rod is key-hole in shape.

   d. Hardened enamel is 50% organic and 50% inorganic.

5. Which of the following is correct regarding dentin?

   a. Dentin formation begins after enamel formation.

   b. Odontoblasts within the dental papilla form dentin.

   c. Dentin is 30% organic and 70% inorganic material.

   d. The dentin of the tooth is laid down all at once and then calcified.

6. Which of the following structures is directly responsible for formation of the cementum?

    a. dental sac

    b. dental papilla

    c. enamel organ

    d. dental lamina

7. Which of the following statements regarding enamel is not correct?

    a. Enamel is the hardest substance in the body.

    b. Enamel has the ability to repair itself.

    c. Enamel is thinner at the cementoenamel junction.

    d. Enamel is whiter at the chewing surface and cusp tips.

8. Which of the following is not correct regarding the periodontal ligament?

    a. The periodontal ligament fibers embed into the cementum of the tooth and lamina dura of the alveolar bone.

    b. The periodontal ligament is located in the space between the alveolar socket and the root of the tooth.

    c. The periodontal ligament is rigid, thus preventing any movement of the tooth during function.

    d. The periodontal ligament carries blood supply to periodontium for nutrition and remodeling.

9. Which of the following is correct regarding the gingiva?

    a. Healthy gingival tissue should be red in color with some swelling.

    b. The free gingiva starts where the gingiva is in contact with the tooth and should be below the cementoenamel junction of the tooth.

    c. The free gingiva is unattached gingiva and is usually 1 to 3 millimeters starting from the margin.

    d. In health, the sulcus of the gingiva should be 3 to 5 millimeters in depth.

10. Which of the following structures marks where the free gingiva ends and the attached gingiva begins?

    a. free marginal groove

    b. epithelial attachment

    c. sulcus

    d. mucogingival junction

CHAPTER APPLICATION

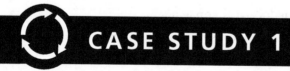

CASE STUDY 1

Ariel is concerned about the staining on her teeth, and she has brought this concern to the dentist's attention. She has noticed the staining for some time, but as yet no one has suggested a cause.

1. Why would the dentist inquire whether tetracycline was taken?

    _____

    _____

    _____

CASE STUDY 2

A young female presents to the office with her mother. The mother is concerned with the appearance of the enamel of the teeth. The mother states that the enamel is soft, and you notice that it has pits. In the life cycle of the tooth, certain developmental disturbances can occur.

1. What may have happened in this case?

_____

_____

2. What are the likely causes of pitting and grooving of tooth surfaces?

_____

_____

3. State the developmental stage at which pitting and grooving most likely occur.

_____

_____

Critical Thinking

1. What occurs in the inner enamel epithelial cells as they mature to become ameloblasts?

_____

_____

_____

_____

_____

2. What is the process that takes place in the formation of enamel?

_____

_____

_____

_____

_____

_____

3. What is the difference between primary, secondary, and tertiary dentin?

_____

_____

_____

_____

_____

_____

_____

_____

_____

_____

_____

_____

_____

_____

CHAPTER 8

Dental Anatomy

SPECIFIC INSTRUCTIONAL OBJECTIVES

The student should strive to meet the following objectives and demonstrate an understanding of the facts and principles presented in this chapter:

1. Use terms presented in this chapter.
2. Describe the types of teeth and their functions.
3. Identify the dental arches, quadrants, and sextants.
4. Discuss the dentition periods.
5. Locate the surfaces of each tooth.
6. Identify line angles, point angles, and divisions into thirds.
7. Recognize anatomic features of teeth.
8. Identify landmarks of a tooth.
9. Discuss the morphology of teeth.
10. Locate maxillary and mandibular anterior teeth landmarks.
11. Compare and contrast the maxillary anterior teeth with the mandibular anterior Teeth.
12. Locate maxillary and mandibular posterior teeth landmarks.
13. Compare and contrast the maxillary posterior teeth with the mandibular posterior teeth.
14. Use the Universal Numbering System when identifying teeth.
15. Compare and contrast primary and permanent anterior teeth.
16. Compare and contrast primary and permanent posterior teeth.

VOCABULARY BUILDER

Matching

Match each term with the appropriate definition.

1. _____ anterior
2. _____ buccal
3. _____ cervical
4. _____ maxillary

a. next to cheek
b. upper arch
c. in the front
d. neck of tooth

5. _____ eruption
6. _____ exfoliate
7. _____ extract
8. _____ dentition

a. tooth removed from mouth
b. tooth entering mouth
c. shedding of tooth
d. set of teeth

9. _____ fossa
10. _____ groove
11. _____ cusp
12. _____ cingulum

a. elevation on lingual of anterior teeth
b. line depression on tooth surface
c. scooped out depression on tooth surface
d. pointed elevation

13. _____ ante
14. _____ dent
15. _____ inter
16. _____ lingua

a. between
b. before
c. tongue
d. teeth

Fill in the Blank

Please fill in the blank with one of the choices provided.

embrasure   distal   tongue

middle   tooth   distal

third

1. The surface of the tooth that is away from the midline is the _____.

2. The _____ surface touches the mesial of the adjacent tooth within the arch.

3. The triangular space near the gingiva between teeth is the _____.

4. The area on the crown of the tooth between the incisal third and the cervical third is called the _____.

CHAPTER REVIEW

True or False

Circle whether the answer is true of false.

1. **T F** A convex surface means that the surface is recessed.

2. **T F** Interproximal surfaces are between adjacent teeth.

3. **T F** The area on the crown of the tooth that is closest to the cutting edge on the anterior tooth is called the incisal third.

4. **T F** The teeth closest to the midline are the canines.

5. **T F** A developmental groove that has an imperfect union where the lobes join is called a fissure.

Multiple Choice

1. The _____ line angle is at almost a 90 degree angle on incisors.

   a. distal–incisal
   b. mesial–incisal

   c. distal–labial
   d. mesial–lingual

2. Which feature of the tooth prevents food trapping between teeth, holds teeth in place, and protects gingival tissue from trauma?

   a. contour
   b. contact

   c. height of contour
   d. embrasure

3. Which tooth has a sharp, pointed cutting surface used to cut and tear food?

   a. incisor
   b. canine

   c. premolar
   d. molar

4. What tooth has the broadest surface with multiple cusps to chew or grind the food?

   a. incisor
   b. canine

   c. premolar
   d. molar

5. The permanent teeth that replace the primary teeth are called _____ teeth.

   a. deciduous
   b. milk teeth

   c. succedaneous
   d. mamelon

6. How many molars are in the permanent dentition?

   a. 3
   b. 6

   c. 12
   d. 16

7. Which type of tooth is only found in the permanent dentition?

   a. incisor
   b. cuspid

   c. premolar
   d. molar

8. The cusp on mandibular molars that is normally the smallest is the _____.

    a. mesio-buccal

    b. disto-buccal

    c. mesio-lingual

    d. disto-lingual

9. Which of the premolars may have two or three cusps?

    a. maxillary first

    b. maxillary second

    c. mandibular first

    d. mandibular second

10. The primary (deciduous) dentition consists of

    a. 32 teeth, 18 in each arch, and 9 in each quadrant.

    b. 20 teeth, 10 in each arch, and 5 in each quadrant.

    c. 16 teeth, 8 in each arch, and 4 in each quadrant.

    d. 12 teeth, 6 in each arch, and 3 in each quadrant.

11. The primary first molar is replaced by an adult

    a. canine.

    b. premolar.

    c. first molar.

    d. lateral.

12. Which are the five surfaces found on an anterior tooth?

    a. mesial, distal, palatal, buccal, and incisal

    b. mesial, distal, lingual, labial, and occlusal

    c. mesial, distal, lingual, labial, and incisal

    d. mesial, distal, palatal, buccal, and occlusal

13. Which tooth has trifurcated roots?

    a. maxillary premolars

    b. maxillary molars

    c. mandibular premolars

    d. mandibular molars

14. Which tooth has bifurcated roots?

    a. maxillary first premolar

    b. maxillary second premolar

    c. mandibular first premolar

    d. mandibular second premolar

15. Which tooth has an oblique ridge?

    a. maxillary premolars

    b. maxillary molars

    c. mandibular premolars

    d. mandibular molars

Matching

Match the following terms with the primary teeth in the following diagram.

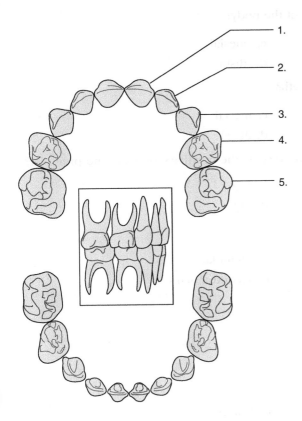

1. _____ ( )

2. _____ ( )

3. _____ ( )

4. _____ ( )

5. _____ ( )

1. canine

2. central incisor

3. first molar

4. second molar

5. lateral incisor

CERTIFICATION REVIEW

1. All of these anatomical features of the maxillary canine are larger and more developed than the mandibular canine EXCEPT

   a. the cingulum.

   b. the cusp.

   c. fossa.

   d. crown length.

2. Which permanent tooth may have a cusp of Carabelli?

   a. mandibular first molar

   b. maxillary first molar

   c. mandibular second molar

   d. maxillary second molar

3. Which of the succedaneous teeth erupt first?

   a. mandibular premolars

   b. mandibular incisors

   c. maxillary molars

   d. maxillary canines

4. How many teeth are in a fully erupted permanent dentition?

    a. 20 teeth   c. 28 teeth

    b. 24 teeth   d. 32 teeth

5. Which surface of a tooth is closest toward the midline of the body?

    a. occlusal   c. mesial

    b. lingual   d. distal

6. Which is the broad chewing surface of the posterior teeth?

    a. occlusal   c. mesial

    b. lingual   d. distal

7. Using the universal numbering system, which symbol represents the maxillary right second premolar?

    a. #4   c. #12

    b. #5   d. #13

8. Which teeth are not found in the primary dentition?

    a. first molars   c. premolars

    b. canines   d second molars

9. Which of these describe incisors?

    1. single rooted

    2. located in the anterior portion of the mouth

    3. have one cusp

    4. have thin sharp edges for cutting

        a. 1, 2   c. 1, 2, 3

        b. 2, 3   d. 1, 2, 4

10. Which of these describe canines?

    1. designed to tear food

    2. have a pointed cusp

    3. referred to as the cornerstones of the dental arch

    4. also referred to a cuspids

        a. 1, 2   c. 1, 2, 4

        b. 2, 3, 4   d. 1, 2, 3, 4

CHAPTER APPLICATION

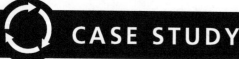

CASE STUDY

The dental assistant explains to Cory's mother that their D. maxillary central incisor needs to be extracted due to severe decay. Cory is 6 years old.

1. When do the D. maxillary central incisors normally exfoliate?

_____

_____

2. At what age do the adult maxillary central incisors normally erupt?

_____

_____

3. For how long will Cory be without front teeth?

_____

_____

4. How will the loss of these teeth affect Cory?

_____

_____

Image Labeling

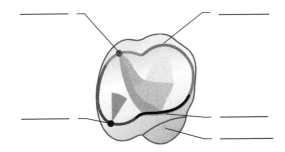

1. What tooth is labeled below?

_____

_____

2. What is the name of the landmark labeled A?

_____

_____

3. What is the name of the landmark labeled B?

_____

_____

4. What is the name of the landmark labeled C?

_____

_____

5. What is the name of the landmark labeled E?

_____

_____

6. On the following figure, identify the tooth by name and its universal numbering system symbol.

_____

_____

_____

_____

_____

CHAPTER 9

Oral Pathology

SPECIFIC INSTRUCTIONAL OBJECTIVES

The student should strive to meet the following objectives and demonstrate an understanding of the facts and principles presented in this chapter:

1. Use terms presented in this chapter.
2. Define oral pathology.
3. Identify the role of the dental assistant in the area of oral pathology.
4. Discuss the methods used to identify a lesion.
5. Define the three phases of inflammation.
6. Identify various lesions based on location.
7. Discuss the dental caries process.
8. Explain the four stages of decay.
9. Summarize the causes of rampant caries.
10. Compare and contrast lesions of the oral cavity caused by biological agents.
11. Differentiate between amelogenesis imperfect and dentinogenesis imperfecta.
12. Compare and contrast anodontia and hypodontia.
13. Compare and contrast fusion and gemination.
14. Differentiate between macrodontia and microdontia.
15. Explain the various anomalies of the tongue.
16. Summarize the lesions produced by chemical agents.
17. Differentiate among the lesions produced by physical agents.
18. Identify the lesions that are caused by hormonal imbalances.
19. Differentiate among the lesions produced by nutritional deficiencies.
20. Compare and contrast between benign and malignant neoplasms.

21. List the common sites for oral cancer.

22. State the warning signs for oral cancer.

23. Compare and contrast leukoplakia and erythroplakia.

24. Discuss the two forms of lichen planus.

25. Discuss the oral lesions related to HIV and AIDS.

26. Explain the importance of oral cancer screening.

27. Outline the steps in a head and neck exam for oral cancer.

28. Outline the steps for a patient self-exam for oral cancer.

29. Compare and contrast the types of diagnostic tools available for oral cancer screening.

30. Compare and contrast patient treatment before, during and after radiation therapy.

VOCABULARY BUILDER

Matching

Match each term with the appropriate definition.

1. _____ erythematous

2. _____ necrotic

3. _____ hyperkeratosis

4. _____ malignant

5. _____ abscess

6. _____ indurated

7. _____ encapsulated

8. _____ mucositis

9. _____ chancre

10. _____ prodromal

a. enclosed by a protective coating or membrane

b. small hard nodular growth; first sign of syphilis

c. collection of purulent exudate or pus

d. reddening of the skin

e. pathologic death of one or more cells

f. growing worse, resisting treatment, threatening to produce death

g. the thickening of the stratum corneum, often associated with a quantitative abnormality of the keratin

h. early symptoms that signify the start of a disease

i. inflammation of a mucous membrane

j. hardened, becoming extremely firm but not as hard as bone

CHAPTER REVIEW

True or False

Choose the best answer.

1. There are three phases to the clinical diagnosis. This includes location, size, and color
   a. Both statements are true.
   b. Both statements are false.
   c. The first statement is true; the second statement is false.
   d. The first statement is false; the second statement is true.

2. Some lesions may be in several lobes or segmented parts and can be said to be lobulated. In such cases, each lobe of the lesion should be measured separately.
   a. Both statements are true.
   b. Both statements are false.
   c. The first statement is true; the second statement is false.
   d. The first statement is false; the second statement is true.

3. Angular cheilitis is caused by a nutritional deficiency of vitamin C. One way to attempt to diagnose the problem is to give the patient the vitamin they are deficient in and see if the lesion goes away.
   a. Both statements are true.
   b. Both statements are false.
   c. The first statement is true; the second statement is false.
   d. The first statement is false; the second statement is true.

4. T F If a lesion is questionable, it is important that the patient return in 4 weeks to see if healing has progressed.

5. T F The amplification phase is the first phase of the inflammatory process, where white blood cells (WBCs) start to fight off the infection using cells called *neutrophils* and *macrophages* to destroy the invading agents.

6. T F The pH of the oral cavity becomes acidic after eating sugary substances or carbohydrate-rich substances.

Multiple Choice

1. What is the surgical removal of a small amount of the suspicious lesion tissue?
   a. etiology
   b. biopsy
   c. orifice
   d. ankylosis

2. Mast cells release this and bring about swelling.
   a. etiology
   b. histamine
   c. antigen
   d. papule

3. Which of the following are diagnostic tools used to evaluate oral pathology?
   a. radiographs
   b. clinical diagnoses
   c. genetic histories
   d. all of the above

4. The dentist reads the radiographs to note which of the following?

    a. absorption

    b. cysts

    c. abscesses

    d. all of the above

5. In the second stage of syphilis, _____ occur(s).

    a. flu-like symptoms

    b. chancre

    c. gumma

    d. nervous system damage

6. _____ is a bacterial infection that first causes painful swelling and later causes an abscess that drains outside of the mouth.

    a. herpes simplex

    b. actinomycosis

    c. herpes labialis

    d. aphthous ulcer

7. Which bacterial disease has three primary stages, with bone and cartilage being destroyed in the final stage?

    a. Hutchinson's disease

    b. mulberry

    c. syphilis

    d. thrush

8. Which developmental disturbance appears as wrinkled, deeply grooved on the dorsal surface on the tongue?

    a. fissured tongue

    b. ankyloglossia

    c. black hairy tongue

    d. bifid tongue

9. Which of the following conditions is a result of a vitamin B complex deficiency and will form a lesion in the corner of the mouth?

    a. *herpes labialis*

    b. herpetic zoster

    c. angular cheilitis

    d. *Candida albicans*

10. Which of the following lesions is classified as below the surface of the oral mucosa?

    a. bulla

    b. pustule

    c. abscess

    d. granuloma

11 A melanotic macule lesion is

    a. a medical term for bruising of the tissue.

    b. a flat pigmented benign spot

    c. small spots colored red or purple.

    d. caused by bleeding in underlying tissues.

12. Which lesion is caused by bleeding from a ruptured blood vessel during an injection of oral anesthetic?

    a. cyst

    b. blister

    c. hematoma

    d. nodule

13. Which of the following lesions is associated with chronic inflammation and appears as a neoplasm filled with granulation tissue?

    a. ecchymosis

    b. granuloma

    c. nodule

    d. purpura

14. Ecchymosis, a medical term for bruising of the tissue, is

    a. even or flat with the surface of the oral mucosa.

    b. above the surface of the oral mucosa.

    c. below the surface of the oral mucosa.

    d. not found on the oral mucosa.

Matching

Match the following lesion consistency and texture to its description.

Term	Definition
1. _____ denuded	a. covered in small multiple bump-like areas
2. _____ fluctuant	b. raw, as in under a blister after it pops and peels, scraped, open wounds
3. _____ papillary	c. fluid filled and moveable
4. _____ corrugated	d. wrinkled, rippled, layered-like appearance

CERTIFICATION REVIEW

1. Which one of the following is not part of a clinical diagnosis?

   a. location
   b. size
   c. history
   d. shape

2. Which of the following is not correct regarding the dental caries process?

   a. Dental caries develops very rapidly, in a matter of days.
   b. Bacteria such as *Mutans streptococci* are found in the biofilm that builds up on teeth.
   c. The biofilm, combined with fermentable carbohydrates, creates metabolic acids.
   d. Dental caries is transmittable from mother or caregiver to a young child.

3. Which of the following is not correct regarding herpes simplex 1 (HSV1) lesions?

   a. Once the lesion heals, the virus enters the latent phase.
   b. The lesion initially appears as clusters of small vesicles.
   c. It is acceptable to treat patients in the active stage of HSV1.
   d. Apthous ulcers usually occur on keratinized tissue.

4. Which of the following is correct regarding amelogenesis imperfecta?

   a. The dentin is softer than normal in amelogenesis imperfect.
   b. Amelogenesis imperfect is not a genetic disorder.
   c. Radiographs show a large pulp chamber.
   d. The soft dentin causes the enamel to chip off.

5. Recurrant apthous ulcers that vary from 8 to 10 mm in size and are commonly seen in the nonkeratinized mucosal surfaces of labial mucosa, buccal mucosa, and floor of the oral cavity are

   a. major.
   b. minor.
   c. herpetiform.
   d. irregular.

6. This lesion is characterized by red, smooth patches where the filiform papillae are not present on the dorsal and lateral surfaces of the tongue.

   a. fissured tongue

   b. bifid tongue

   c. ankyloglossia

   d. geographic tongue

7. Which of the following causes a white, corrugated, hyperkeratinized, wrinkled lesion in the buccal vestibule?

   a. chewing tobacco

   b. black hairy tongue

   c. gingival hyperplasia

   d. aspirin burn

8. Which of the following causes the filiform papillae on the dorsum of the tongue to become elongated because of a build-up of stain by food, tobacco, and chromogenic bacteria?

   a. chewing tobacco

   b. black hairy tongue

   c. gingival hyperplasia

   d. aspirin burn

9. Which of the following benign neoplasms has a soap-bubble appearance and is most commonly associated with the dentigerous cyst of an unerupted tooth?

   a. pleomorphic adenoma

   b. papilloma

   c. ameloblastoma

   d. ranula

10. Which of the following is the most common intraoral site for squamous cell carcinoma?

    a. tongue

    b. floor of the oral cavity

    c. lip

    d. exposed skin

CHAPTER APPLICATION

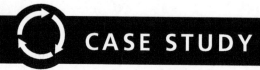

CASE STUDY

Max is scheduled for a recall appointment with the hygienist. Before Max sees the hygienist, the dental assistant prepares to take radiographs and does an intraoral evaluation. A lesion is seen in the oral vestibule of the lower anterior between the lip and the teeth. The patient does report using smokeless tobacco.

1. Describe a typical lesion caused by smokeless tobacco.

   _____

   _____

   _____

2. What is another name for this lesion?

_____

_____

_____

3. This lesion is considered premalignant. Which type of carcinoma has been documented with this type of lesion?

_____

_____

_____

4. If the patient discontinues use of smokeless tobacco after patient education is performed, what are some signs that the lesion is healing?

_____

_____

_____

Critical Thinking

1. A dental assistant does not diagnose, but may alert the dentist to, abnormal conditions in the mouth. After an injection, what should the dental assistant monitor the injection site for? What is the cause?

_____

_____

_____

2. Oral piercings are a means of self-expression and body art. The number of people who are seeking oral piercing is on the rise. List areas of the oral cavity where an oral piercing may be placed, and describe one of the most serious side effects of piercing.

_____

_____

_____

3. Bulimic patients go through bouts of binge eating and self-induced vomiting. What are some signs that may indicate this eating disorder?

_____

_____

_____

4. What lesion is a benign tumor of connective tissue cells that is not a "true" neoplasm and is usually caused by continuous irritation to an area that causes the tissue to grow?

_____

_____

_____

5. What are the two types of carcinoma that are of most concern in dentistry, and which one accounts for most cases of oral cancer?

_____

_____

_____

6. What are the four most common sites of oral cancer in order from most common to least common?

_____

_____

_____

Preclinical Dental Sciences

Microbiology

The student should strive to meet the following objectives and demonstrate an understanding of the facts and principles presented in this chapter:

1. Use terms presented in this chapter.

2. Explain why the study of microbiology is important to the dental assistant.

3. Identify the early pioneers in microbiology and their contributions to current understanding of microorganism.

4. Discuss the nature of the disease process.

5. Discuss the major groups of microorganism, prions, and normal flora.

6. Distinguish bacterial, viral, protozoal, fungal, rickettsial, algal, and prion diseases.

7. Discuss the harmful effects of normal flora.

8. Describe the body's resistance to disease.

9. Explain types of immunity and vaccines.

10. Discuss the role of epidemiology in controlling communicable diseases.

VOCABULARY BUILDER

Fill in the Blank

Please fill in the blank with one of the choices provided.

vaccine	carrier	acute
virus	AIDS	body

1. When a condition has a rapid and severe onset, it is _____.

2. _____ is a disease of the immune system primarily caused through sexual contact or sharing contaminated needles with infected individuals.

3. A _____ is a person that harbors an infectious agent of a disease and capable of transmitting the disease.

4. A _____ is introduced into the body to induce immunity.

5. A _____ is a microorganism that replicates in living cells.

Matching

Match each term with the appropriate definition.

1. _____ antiobiotic
2. _____ biofilm
3. _____ pathogen
4. _____ phagocyte
5. _____ antigen

a. disease-producing microorganism
b. mass of bacteria growing on teeth
c. ingest foreign bacteria disease-producing microorganism
d. treats bacterial infections
e. stimulates production of antibody

6. _____ anti
7. _____ path
8. _____ hepat
9. _____ phago
10. _____ gen

a. liver
b. to produce
c. disease
d. against
e. devour

11. _____ artificially acquired immunity
12. _____ antimicrobial
13. _____ innate immunity
14. _____ antibody
15. _____ biofilm

a. dental plaque
b. body produces own antibodies
c. inhibits/kills pathogenic microorganisms
d. neutralizes pathogenic bacteria/viruses
e. resistance to disease as part of natural biologic makeup

CHAPTER REVIEW

Matching

Match each term with the appropriate definition.

1. _____ Antony van Leeuwenhoek
2. _____ Louis Pasteur
3. _____ Joseph Lister
4. _____ John Tyndall

5. _____ Robert Koch
6. _____ Hans Christian Gram

a. developed staining to classify types of bacteria
b. isolated organisms causing anthrax, TB, and cholera
c. first to observe microorganisms through microscope
d. discovered process to kill germs; known as Father of Microbiology
e. discovered bacteria in air
f. practiced antiseptic surgery

Multiple Choice

1. The study of microorganisms is called

   a. pathogens.

   b. microbiology.

   c. bacteria.

   d. virus.

2. When a specific type of bacteria causes a specific disease, it is called the _____ agent.

   a. antibody

   b. virus

   c. spore

   d. etiologic

3. _____ bacteria are destroyed in the presence of oxygen.

   a. Aerobic

   b. Anaerobic

   c. Facultative anaerobic

   d. Sporulating

4. Under a microscope, _____ bacteria will appear rod shaped.

   a. cocci

   b. spirilla

   c. vibrios

   d. bacilli

5. Under a microscope, _____ bacteria will appear round or bead shaped.

   a. cocci

   b. spirilla

   c. vibrios

   d. bacilli

6. Bacteria grown in colonies or clusters like grapes are called

   a. diplococci.

   b. staphylococci.

   c. streptococci.

   d. bacilli.

7. Name the group of bacteria that have been known to contribute to dental caries and endocarditis, as well as lead to pneumonia or rheumatic fever.

   a. staphylococcal

   b. streptococcal

   c. bacilli

   d. protozoa

8. Protozoa and bacteria together cause a dental condition called _____ that is found in the inflamed tissue around the tooth.

   a. dental decay

   b. calculus/tartar

   c. periodontal disease

   d. candidiasis

9. _____ are the smallest microorganisms known to date and can be visualized only under an electron microscope.

   a. Bacteria

   b. Tinea

   c. Typhus

   d. Viruses

10. Which of the following diseases are caused by a virus?

    1. measles

    2. typhus

    3. malaria

       a. 1, 3, 6

       b. 1, 4, 6

    4. chicken pox

    5. Creutzfeldt–Jakob syndrome

    6. hepatitis

       c. 1, 2, 3

       d. 2, 3, 6

11. Which viral disease is usually associated with infections of the lips, mouth, and face?

    a. herpetic whitlow

    b. conjunctivitis

    c. herpes simplex virus type 2

    d. herpes simplex virus type 1

12. _____ (a virus) is extremely contagious and can spread by direct contact with the lesion or the fluid from the lesion.

    a. HIV

    b. hepatitis C

    c. herpes simplex

    d. hepatitis B

13. A(n) _____ is a group of symptoms that characterizes a disease.

    a. syndrome

    b. etiologic agent

    c. spore

    d. bacterium

14. As its final line of defense, the body forms _____ to produce immunity against a foreign substance.

    a. antigens

    b. antibodies

    c. antitoxins

    d. pathogens

15. If immunity develops as a result of exposure to a pathogen, the immunity is called

    a. innate.

    b. passively acquired.

    c. artificially acquired.

    d. actively acquired.

16. An individual who has the ability to resist pathogens is called

    a. an allergen.

    b. hypersensitive.

    c. immune.

    d. erythemic.

Matching

Match each type of microorganism with a disease.

Microorganism

1. _____ bacteria

2. _____ rickettsiae

3. _____ fungus

4. _____ virus

Disease

a. MMR, influenza

b. *Candida albicans*

c. Typhus

d. TB, DPT

Match each of the following diseases with its respective infection.

Disease

1. _____ herpes simplex virus type 1

2. _____ herpes simplex virus type 2

3. _____ hepatitis B

4. _____ HIV

Infection

a. serum hepatitis

b. infection of CD4 T-cells

c. infections of lips, mouth, and face

d. associated with genital area

CERTIFICATION REVIEW

1. Which of the following is the most infectious bloodborne pathogen likely to be encountered in the dental workplace?

   a. hepatitis B

   b. HIV

   c. tuberculosis

   d. prion disease

2. Which hepatitis virus is NOT transmitted by bloodborne bacteria?

   a. A

   b. B

   c. C

   d. D

3. Which virus was declared a pandemic in 2020, resulting in dental offices being mandated to temporarily close to all but urgent and emergency procedures?

   a. ebola

   b. Zika

   c. coronavirus

   d. H1N1

4. Which of the following oral diseases may be transmitted with or without the presence of an active lesion?

   a. candidiasis

   b. herpes simplex

   c. dental caries

   d. periodontitis

5. What type of bacteria requires oxygen to survive?

   a. anaerobic

   b. aerobic

   c. facultative anaerobic

   d. facultative aerobic

6. Which is highly resistant to dying and is used to test sterilization methods?

   a. parasites

   b. spores

   c. facultative anaerobes

   d. viruses

7. Which is a highly contagious bacterial infection contracted through inhalation of droplets from an infected individual?

   a. MRSA

   b. tuberculosis

   c. tetanus

   d. shingles

8. Which immunity occurs after contact with a disease-causing antigen?

   a. innate immunity
   b. naturally acquired active immunity
   c. naturally acquired passive immunity
   d. artificially acquired immunity

9. Which immunizations are highly recommended by the CDC for health care personnel?

   a. hepatitis C, HZT, H1N1, and influenza
   b. MMR, hepatitis C, shingles, and TB
   c. tetanus, MRSA, hepatitis B, and ebola
   d. hepatitis B, influenza, varicella zoster, and MMR

10. What term is used to describe infectious diseases that spread over several countries, affecting a large number of people?

    a. pandemic
    b. outbreak
    c. epidemic
    d. panoramic

CHAPTER APPLICATION

CASE STUDY 1

Bloodborne diseases are of major concern to the dental assistant. One of these diseases is transmitted directly through blood-contaminated body fluids.

1. Name the five different types of viral hepatitis. Which is of major concern to dental personnel?

   _____

   _____

   _____

2. Name a high-risk behavior for acquiring hepatitis B, HIV, and AIDS.

   _____

   _____

   _____

CASE STUDY 2

Dental assistants must protect themselves against bacteria and also from the patient transmitting bacteria. One of the most common bacterial diseases infecting humans is strep throat.

1. Name the bacterial type that causes strep throat.

_____

_____

_____

2. List the symptoms of strep throat.

_____

_____

_____

3. Name some of the conditions this bacterium can cause.

_____

_____

_____

Critical Thinking

1. Ferdinand Julius Cohn, a biologist, studied the life cycle of *Bacillus*. Why have his findings had such an impact on how dental offices perform sterilization?

_____

_____

_____

2. Pasteur discovered a method of using an artificially generated weak form of a disease to fight the disease or prevent its occurrence. His work laid the foundation for many of these now being produced. Name this disease-fighting development.

_____

_____

_____

3. Individually, the health care worker must take action to enhance their ability to resist pathogens and thus disease.

   a. What vaccinations should the dental assistant have?

_____

_____

b. What diseases should NOT be treated in the dental office when in the infectious stage?

_____

_____

_____

c. What bloodborne diseases are of concern to the dental assistant?

_____

_____

CHAPTER 11

Infection Control

SPECIFIC INSTRUCTIONAL OBJECTIVES

At the completion of this chapter, you will be able to meet these objectives:

1. Use terms presented in this chapter.
2. Describe the five steps to achieving asepsis in the dental office.
3. Identify when to perform hand hygiene.
4. Outline the steps in the three hand hygiene techniques used in dentistry.
5. State the purpose of each component of personal protective equipment (PPE).
6. Compare and contrast among the types of gloves used in dentistry.
7. Describe the steps in donning and doffing personal protective equipment (PPE).
8. Define sanitization.
9. Differentiate among housekeeping surfaces and clinical contact surfaces.
10. Compare and contrast precleaning and disinfecting of contaminated surfaces.
11. Discuss clinical surface barriers.
12. Discuss waste disposal.
13. Describe the recommended layout of the instrument processing area.
14. Describe the seven steps in instrument processing for contaminated instruments.
15. Discuss the purpose of the ultrasonic cleaner.
16. Outline the steps in operating an ultrasonic cleaner.
17. Discuss the steps in managing a contaminated patient tray in the sterilization area.
18. Define disinfection.
19. Compare and contrast the three categories of instruments.
20. Compare and contrast among the different levels of disinfectants.

21. Discuss the disinfection process of clinical contact surfaces.

22. Discuss the disinfection process of transfer surfaces.

23. Discuss the process of disinfecting contaminated instruments.

24. Identify the factors that can impact disinfectant efficiency.

25. Discuss the importance of disinfecting waterlines.

26. Discuss the importance of disinfecting dental vacuum hoses.

27. Discuss the importance of sterilization.

28. Compare and contrast among the various methods of sterilization.

29. Outline the steps in operating a steam autoclave.

30. Discuss the process of handpiece sterilization.

31. Describe the factors that can impact sterilization.

32. Compare and contrast the methods of monitoring sterilization.

33. Describe the roles of the various agencies in providing guidelines for infection control in dentistry.

34. Define standard precautions.

35. Discuss the Bloodborne Pathogens Standard.

36. Discuss the Hazard Communication Standards.

VOCABULARY BUILDER

Matching

Match each term with the appropriate definition.

1. _____ asepsis

2. _____ bioburden

3. _____ cross-contamination

4. _____ culture

5. _____ dermatitis

6. _____ efficacy

7. _____ ergonomics

8. _____ fungicidal

9. _____ heterotrophic

10. _____ planktonic

a. capable of destroying viruses

b. determining if sterilizer is effective with a spore strip

c. penetration of liquids and pathogens through minute openings in latex membranes

d. passage by needle puncture

e. microorganisms floating in water

f. capable of destroying mycobacterium tuberculosis

g. occurring after exposure to a disease

h. skin inflammation

i. presence of microorganisms or their toxins in tissues

j. absence of disease-producing microorganisms

(Continues)

11. _____ percutaneous

12. _____ post-exposure

13. _____ sanitize

14. _____ sepsis

15. _____ sporicidal

16. _____ sterilant

17. _____ sterile

18. _____ tuberculocidal

19. _____ virucidal

20. _____ wicking

k. transmission of disease-carrying microorganisms from one area or person to another

l. sterilizing agent

m. capable of killing spores

n. to make free from dirt or germs

o. capable of destroying fungi

p. able to produce a desired result

q. science related to work areas for efficiency

r. number of contaminating bacteria on a nonsterile surface

s. free from all living microorganisms

t. organism that obtains food and energy from organic substances

CHAPTER REVIEW

True or False

Circle whether the answer is true or false.

1. **T   F**   Asepsis means the creation of an environment free of disease-causing microorganisms.

2. **T   F**   Employers must protect their employees from exposure to blood and OPIM during the time when employees are at work.

3. **T   F**   OSHA states that when removing protective clothing, special care is to be taken with items that are considered potentially infectious.

4. **T   F**   Low-level disinfection will kill bacterial spores.

5. **T   F**   A heat-sensitive tape used to identify when materials have been sterilized is a type of biological monitor.

Multiple Choice

1. In 1992, OSHA established the Bloodborne Pathogens Standard. It mandates that facilities must do which of the following?

   1. provide infection control training manuals
   2. protect workers from infectious hazards
   3. protect workers from chemical hazards
   4. protect workers from physical hazards

   a. 1, 2

   b. 1, 2, 3

   c. 2, 3

   d. 1, 2, 3, 4

2. What cycle is perpetuated when pathogens are allowed to pass from dentist to patient or from patient to dentist?

   a. material safety data

   b. cross-contamination

   c. pathogens standard

   d. standard exposure

3. One of the primary concerns of handwashing is to remove the _____ microorganisms because they constitute the group that includes hepatitis.

   a. transient
   b. causative

   c. bloodborne
   d. saliva

4. During handwashing a generous lather is produced by rubbing hands together for how many seconds?

   a. 60
   b. 30

   c. 15
   d. 90

5. Barriers that prevent potential pathogens encountered during patient care from gaining access to dental personnel include which of the following?

   1. safety data sheets (SDS)
   2. EPA
   3. regulations
   4. gloves
   5. mask
   6. eyewear
      a. 1, 2, 3
      b. 4, 5, 6

      c. 1, 4, 5
      d. 2, 3, 5

6. Which type of gloves are used for patient treatment whenever the dental assistant anticipates contact with saliva or blood?

   a. examination
   b. overgloves

   c. utility
   d. knitted

7. Which of the following are recommended for use by dental assistants as protection from aerosol mists during the Covid-19 pandemic?

   a. overgloves
   b. N95 masks

   c. rubber dams
   d. lead aprons

8. Concerning the asepsis requirement, some surfaces do not lend themselves to the use of barriers. Those surfaces will need to be _____.

   a. suctioned
   b. sterilized

   c. autoclaved
   d. disinfected

9. According to EPA-ratings, which disinfection level will kill most bacterial spores?

   a. high
   b. intermediate

   c. low
   d. holding

10. Which of the following EPA-registered disinfectants is considered to be a high-level disinfectant?

    a. alcohol
    b. glutaraldehyde

    c. iodophor
    d. sodium hypochlorite

11. Which of the following EPA-registered disinfectants is considered an intermediate-level disinfectant?

    a. alcohol
    b. hydrogen peroxide

    c. glutaraldehyde
    d. iodophor

12. Which device that uses sound waves that vibrate and create invisible bubbles in a special solution to clean debris from dental instruments?

    a. sterilizer

    b. autoclave

    c. ultrasonic cleaner

    d. holding bath

13. Which process destroys all forms of microorganisms?

    a. disinfection

    b. asepsis

    c. sterilization

    d. sanitization

14. If immersion sterilization is used, what is the minimum number of hours the instruments are placed in the disinfecting solution ensure that all microorganisms are destroyed?

    a. 1

    b. 5

    c. 10

    d. 3

15. Which is the most accurate way to assess sterilization?

    a. cavitation

    b. biological test

    c. cleaning

    d. sanitizing

CERTIFICATION REVIEW

1. What is the purpose of placing loose and contaminated instruments in an ultrasonic cleaner?

    a. disinfection and cleaning

    b. disinfection only

    c. cleaning only

    d. Remove any large particles.

2. According to OSHA, how long should sterilization monitoring records be maintained?

    a. They do not need to be maintained.

    b. for 10 years after the batch was sterilized

    c. for 6 years after the autoclave was monitored

    d. according to state and local regulations

3. Which of the following is correct regarding semicritical instruments?

    a. Semicritical instruments contact only mucous membranes and nonintact skin.

    b. Semicritical instruments include blood pressure cuffs and radiology machine heads.

    c. Semicritical instruments may be disinfected with an intermediate-level EPA-registered hospital disinfectant with tuberculocidal claim prior to reuse on another patient.

    d. None of the above are correct.

4. Which of the following is correct regarding intermediate-level disinfectants?

    a. Intermediate-level disinfectants may be used for sterilization of critical instruments that are sensitive to heat.

    b. Intermediate-level disinfectants are recommended on clinical contact surfaces and noncritical surfaces soiled with visible blood.

    c. Intermediate-level disinfectants destroy all microorganisms except high numbers of bacterial endospores.

    d. Intermediate-level disinfectants include glutaraldehyde.

5. Which of the following is correct regarding dry heat sterilization?

   a. One type of dry heat sterilizer is a static air sterilizer.
   b. Dry heat sterilizers work at temperatures lower than that of steam sterilizers.
   c. The dry heat sterilizers cause rusting and corrosion of some instruments.
   e. Instrument packages can be stacked in a dry heat sterilizer, allowing for more efficient sterilization.

6. Which of the following is correct regarding handpiece sterilization?

   a. All handpieces should be placed in the ultrasonic solution prior to sterilization.
   b. All handpieces require lubrication prior to sterilization.
   c. Only steam or chemical vapor sterilization is recommended for handpieces.
   d. Handpieces are not exposed to blood or saliva and therefore do not need to be sterilized.

7. Which of the following is correct regarding process integrators?

   a. Process integrators do not indicate sterility.
   b. Process integrators are used externally on sterilization packaging.
   c. Process integrators are considered to be single parameter instruments as they respond to temperature.
   d. Autoclave tape with color change markers is an example of a process integrator.

8. Which of the following is not correct regarding biological monitoring?

   a. Biological monitoring is also known as spore testing.
   b. Biological monitoring is the preferred method of sterilization monitoring.
   c. Biological monitoring is the only way to monitor that sterilization has occurred.
   d. The CDC, the ADA, and OSAP recommend monthly biological monitoring of sterilization equipment.

9. Which of the following statements is correct regarding waste disposal in a dental office?

   a. All waste in a dental office is considered regulated waste.
   b. Containers for medically regulated waste do not need to be specifically identified.
   c. Any disposable item that has been in contact with blood or saliva is considered to be regulated medical waste.
   d. Regulated medical waste is soaked in blood or saliva and capable of releasing blood or saliva during handling.

10. Which of the following is not a correct statement regarding the use of examination gloves in the dental office?

    a. Gloves are used by the dental health care worker to help protect the worker from pathogens.
    b. Gloves are used by the dental health care worker to help prevent pathogenic microorganisms from being transmitted from the worker to the patient.
    c. Gloves are used by the dental health care worker to reduce contamination of the DHCW's hands by organisms transmitted from one patient to another.
    d. Gloves are a substitute for hand hygiene since the gloves protect the hands of the dental health care worker from contamination.

CHAPTER APPLICATION

CASE STUDY 1

Lisa is a new employee in a dental office. A review of OHSA office compliance instructions discussed PPEs and sharps containers. Several notices had been given to the office regarding the use (wearing in/out of the office) and disposal of the uniform gowns that had been provided (a uniform service was to have been provided and was not). The sharps container was overflowing, and no new replacements had arrived. Observation and how to report noncompliance are contained within the written exposure plan.

1. Which regulating body enforces the requirement that employers protect their employees from blood and OPIM during the time when employees are at work?

   _____

   _____

   _____

2. What standard indicates that every facility must provide PPE?

   _____

   _____

   _____

CASE STUDY 2

Pathogens can travel from personnel to patients. Routes of microbial transmission for most microorganisms can exist and can be missed. Thus, the dental assistant is the primary caretaker of infection control practices.

1. List the three possible routes of microbial transmission.

   _____

   _____

   _____

2. What should the dental assistant do to fight off pathogens encountered due to the close proximity of patients during dental treatment?

   _____

   _____

   _____

3. What is one of the most important ways to prevent the transfer of microorganisms from one person or object to another person?

   _____

   _____

   _____

✗ Critical Thinking

1. What are the factors that can impact the efficiency of a disinfectant?

_____

_____

2. Who establishes regulations for infection control in the dental office?

_____

_____

_____

3. What is OPIM? Describe the role of OPIM.

_____

_____

_____

4. What are the OSHA recommendations for PPE for dental health care workers during the Covid-19 pandemic?

CHAPTER 12

Management of Hazardous Materials

SPECIFIC INSTRUCTIONAL OBJECTIVES

At the completion of this chapter, you will be able to meet these objectives:

1. Use terms presented in this chapter.
2. Identify the scope of the OSHA Bloodborne Pathogens Standard.
3. Describe the components of the OSHA Bloodborne Pathogens Standard.
4. Identify equipment to safeguard employees against injury.
5. Discuss requirements for work site safety.
6. Describe the employee training that is required to meet the OSHA standard for hazardous chemicals.
7. Explain the purpose of OSHA's Hazardous Communication Standard (HCS).
8. Identify the three major changes of the HCS to align with the *Globally Harmonized System of Classification and Labeling of Chemicals (GHS)*.
9. Describe the purpose of safety data sheet manuals.
10. Describe the required format of the new safety data sheets.
11. Identify the nine HCS pictograms.
12. Discuss the rationale for fire extinguishers.
13. Discuss the rationale for an evacuation plan.

VOCABULARY BUILDER

Matching

Match each term with the appropriate definition.

1. _____ Needlestick Safety and Prevention Act

2. _____ Exposure Control Plan

3. _____ needleless systems

4. _____ engineering and work practice controls

5. _____ parenteral

6. _____ Globally Harmonized System of Classification and Labeling of Chemicals

7. _____ Safety Data Sheet

a. office policies and procedures that prevent or reduce the risk of disease transmission between dental office personnel, their families, patients, and the community

b. the physical equipment and mechanical devices that employers provide to safeguard and protect employees at work

c. such devices as a jet injection system or an IV medication system in which a port is used instead of a needle

d. passed by U.S. Congress and directed OSHA to revise its bloodborne pathogens standard

e. a means of piercing mucous membranes on the skin barrier through such events as needlesticks, cuts, and abrasions

f. summaries that provide information about the potential hazards of a product as well as safety measures

g. chemicals and materials are classified and labeled the same way internationally, regardless of where the chemicals are manufactured, sold, or used.

CHAPTER REVIEW

Multiple Choice

1. Dental office employees need to know and comply with the OSHA safety standards. Which of the following is not the subject of an OSHA safety standard?

   a. employee training
   b. labeling/SDS
   c. housekeeping/laundry
   d. ADA

2. The physical equipment and mechanical devices that employers provide to safeguard and protect employees are known as

   a. SDS.
   b. engineering/work practice controls.
   c. housekeeping/laundry.
   d. labeling.

3. A means of piercing mucous membranes or the skin barrier through such events as needlesticks, cuts, and abrasions.

   a. OPIM
   b. parenteral
   c. synovial
   d. biohazardous

4. Which of the following would not go into the sharps container?

   a. orthodontic wire
   b. contaminated needles
   c. surgical knives or blades
   d. rubber dam

5. The sharps container must meet strict standards. Which of the following descriptors is not part of the sharps standard?

   a. labeled

   b. leakproof

   c. wide-mouth opening

   d. puncture resistant

6. If an occupational exposure occurs for any employee, which of the following is (are) required?

   a. The employee must report the incident immediately.

   b. Employer must immediately provide medical evaluation and follow-up.

   c. Medical evaluation and follow-up are made available to the employee at no cost.

   d. all of the above

7. Documentation of an exposure incident must include testing for

   a. tetanus.

   b. MMR.

   c. HBV.

   d. TB.

8. If employees choose to decline testing after an exposure incident, they can delay testing up to how many days?

   a. 90

   b. 60

   c. 30

   d. 28

9. A post-exposure prophylaxis is provided according to the current recommendations of (the)

   a. OSHA.

   b. U.S. Public Health Service.

   c. CDC.

   d. ADA.

10. In accordance with OSHA's standard on access to employee exposure and medical records, the employer must maintain employee records for how many year(s)?

    a. 15

    b. 24

    c. 1

    d. 30

11. Gloves that are contaminated with blood are required to go into

    a. regular waste.

    b. a biohazard container.

    c. the laundry.

    d. a leakproof sharps container.

12. These regulations are intended to ensure a safe work environment regarding the risks of using hazardous chemicals.

    a. ADA

    b. EPA

    c. OSHA

    d. Bloodborne

13. Within how many days of employment, employee training must occur regarding the identification of hazardous chemicals and the use of personal protective equipment (PPE).

    a. 90

    b. 15

    c. 30

    d. 60

14. Under the 2001 revision to OSHA's Bloodborne Pathogen Standard, the employer must maintain a sharps injury log. This log must contain the following incident information

    1. reference to minutes of training

    2. description of injury type

    3. recommendations to employees from patients

    4. brand of device involved

5. description of the act
6. location of the act

   a. 1, 3, 5, 6

   b. 2, 3, 4, 5

   c. 2, 4, 5, 6

   d. 1, 4, 5, 6

15. The employer may be required to complete OSHA Form 200 (Log and Summary of Occupational Injuries and Illnesses) if they have over how many employees?

   a. 5

   b. 10

   c. 15

   d. 20

16. The assistant must wear which gloves while cleaning contaminated surfaces?

   a. latex treatment gloves

   b. nitrile latex gloves

   c. utility gloves

   d. over gloves

Matching

Match the National Fire Protection Association's warning to the appropriate color.

1. _____ health hazard

2. _____ fire hazard

3. _____ reactivity or stability of a chemical

4. _____ PPE needed when using the chemical

   a. blue

   b. yellow

   c. white

   d. red

CERTIFICATION REVIEW

Multiple Choice

1. The availability of the exposure control plan is the responsibility of who?

   a. the employee

   b. the employer

   c. the office manager

   d. the receptionist

2. Which of these is not included in the evacuation plan?

   a. mounted fire extinguishers

   b. exit routes

   c. team leader

   d. diagram of the evacuation route

3. OSHA requires that employees receive training about the risks of using hazardous chemicals how often after the initial training?

   a. monthly

   b. annually

   c. biannually

   d. biennially

4. Summaries that provide information about the potential hazards of a product as well as safety measures are kept in a

   a. safety data sheet.

   b. exposure control plan.

   c. hazardous communication standard.

   d. globally Harmonized System of Classification and Labeling of Chemicals.

5. Piercing a mucous membrane with a human bite is which of the following modes of disease transmission?

    a. skin

    b. mucous membrane

    c. parenteral

    d. indirect

6. According to OSHA, the exposure control plan must be

    a. updated every 6 months.

    b. available in a digital format.

    c. written and updated annually.

    d. updated by the office manager.

7. If the SDS is not available in the office for a given material, what should be done?

    a. Request it from the manufacturer.

    b. Use the material with caution.

    c. Use the material and review the SDS once the manufacturer supplies it.

    d. SDS is not necessary to use a material.

8. The SDS is part of OSHA's

    a. Bloodborne Pathogen Standard.

    b. Hazardous Communication Standard.

    c. Engineering Practice Control Plan.

    d. Work and Site Safety Standard.

9. Engineering and work practice controls include

    a. puncture resistant sharps containers.

    b. laundry on-site.

    c. syringes with a sliding sheath.

    d. jet injection system.

10. The employer must provide the employee with a copy of the evaluating health care professional's opinion within how many days?

    a. 5

    b. 10

    c. 15

    d. 20

CHAPTER APPLICATION

CASE STUDY 1

It is a busy day at the office. The dental assistant disassembles the local anesthetic syringe while wearing patient treatment gloves. While unscrewing the needle, the dental assistant gets a needle stick with the contaminated needle. They notice that the needle somehow came out the side of the cap, most likely during the recapping process.

1. What steps should the dentist take when notifying the source, if known?

    _____

    _____

    _____

    _____

2. What steps should the dental assistant who had the needle stick follow?

_____

_____

_____

_____

3. Who pays the cost for testing?

_____

_____

4. What could have been done to prevent this injury?

_____

_____

Critical Thinking

1. Contaminated syringe sharps injuries occur most frequently during postoperative handling of the anesthetic syringe. What recommendations are made by OSHA regarding needle disposal?

_____

_____

_____

2. How does OSHA define occupational exposure?

_____

_____

_____

_____

3. What is involved in maintaining a hazardous communication program?

_____

_____

_____

_____

_____

_____

_____

_____

_____

CHAPTER 13

The Special Needs and Medically Compromised Patient

SPECIFIC INSTRUCTIONAL OBJECTIVES

At the completion of this chapter, you will be able to meet these objectives:

1. Use the terms presented in this chapter.

2. Differentiate between developmental and acquired disabilities.

3. Define special needs, the Americans with Disability Act (ADA) and a barrier free environment.

4. Summarize the special care for the patient with disabilities.

5. Describe one and two person wheelchair transfers.

6. Discuss dental management of the patient with a sensory disability.

7. Describe potential behavior of a patient with intellectual and developmental disabilities.

8. Describe oral findings of a patient with intellectual and developmental disabilities.

9. Discuss the effects of aging and dental management of the older patient.

10. Describe the cause, characteristics of disorders and diseases that define a patient who is medically compromised.

11. Describe the dental management of disorders and diseases that define a patient who is medically compromised.

VOCABULARY BUILDER

Matching

Match each term with the appropriate definition.

1. _____ cyan
2. _____ -osis
3. _____ -itis
4. _____ hypo-
5. _____ -emia

a. inflammation
b. condition of blood
c. blue
d. condition
e. decreases

6. _____ steno
7. _____ tachy
8. _____ -oma
9. _____ psycho-
10. _____ scler

a. hard
b. narrow, close
c. mental processes
d. accelerated
e. tumor

11. _____ pallor
12. _____ phobia
13. _____ anomaly
14. _____ hypoxia
15. _____ anoxia

a. deficiency of oxygen
b. irrational fear
c. deviation from normal
d. without oxygen
e. loss of color of the face

Fill in the Blank

Please fill in the blank with one of the choices provided.

atrophy   tachycardia   heart attack

jaundice   teratogens   blood

1. The assistant notices a yellowing of the patient's skin. They would note the presence of _____ on the patient's chart.

2. _____ occurs when conditions involving a progressive degeneration of cells results in a wasting away of an organ.

3. The patient's medical record indicates that the patient previously experienced a myocardial infarction. This also known as a _____.

4. The patient complained of an excessively rapid heartbeat during the new patient examination. The dentist instructed the assistant to note the presence of _____.

5. Due to the presence of _____ during the mother's pregnancy the baby was born with birth defects.

CHAPTER REVIEW

True or False

Select the best answer.

1. **T F** Special consideration when receiving dental treatment is necessary for patients with special needs and those who are medically compromised.

2. **T F** The Americans with Disabilities Act prohibits discrimination against a person with a disability who is seeking services, including dental services.

3. Title 3 of the law requires dental offices to make modifications to provide access for patients with disabilities. The offices halls should allow for a 360-degree turn in a wheelchair.

   a. Both statements are true.
   b. Both statements are false.
   c. The first statement is true; the second statement is false.
   d. The first statement is false; the second statement is true.

4. Early morning appointments are best for persons with disabilities. If the patient becomes uncooperative, the appointment should be terminated.

   a. Both statements are true.
   b. Both statements are false.
   c. The first statement is true; the second statement is false.
   d. The first statement is false; the second statement is true.

5. Body wraps may be necessary for patients who have extreme spasticity. Those with severe medical or movement problems may require treatment in a hospital.

   a. Both statements are true.
   b. Both statements are false.
   c. The first statement is true; the second statement is false.
   d. The first statement is false; the second statement is true.

6. **T F** Dental treatment can be managed in the wheelchair for patients on a ventilator or paralyzed.

7. Standardized intelligence tests are used to measure intellectual function. An intellectual disability is referred to as a mild cognitive disorder when patients have an IQ range of 20–34.

   a. Both statements are true.
   b. Both statements are false.
   c. The first statement is true; the second statement is false.
   d. The first statement is false; the second statement is true.

8. A pregnant person's oral health can affect the general health of her baby. Pregnancy causes hormonal changes that may result in gingivitis, periodontitis, and caries.

   a. Both statements are true.
   b. Both statements are false.
   c. The first statement is true; the second statement is false.
   d. The first statement is false; the second statement is true.

9. One of the fastest growing populations seeking dental care is the over 65 years of age. The dental team should expect to see greater tooth loss due to aging.

   a. Both statements are true.
   b. Both statements are false.
   c. The first statement is true; the second statement is false.
   d. The first statement is false; the second statement is true.

10. Hypertension is a risk factor for cerebral vascular accident (CVA). Stroke is the layman's term for a CVA.

   a. Both statements are true.
   b. Both statements are false.
   c. The first statement is true; the second statement is false.
   d. The first statement is false; the second statement is true.

Multiple Choice

1. Which oral findings may be present for a patient over 65 years old?

   a. missing teeth, increased periodontal infections
   b. damaging oral habits, increased dental disease
   c. thinning oral mucosa, possible osteoporosis, gingival recession
   d. increased disease due to decreased immune function, enlarged tongue and tonsils

2. Which disability may involve fissured lips and tongue, macroglossia, mouth breathing, an open bite and problems with swallowing?

   a. multiple sclerosis
   b. Down syndrome
   c. cerebral palsy
   d. amyotrophic lateral sclerosis (ALS)

3. During the two person wheelchair transfer, where should the wheelchair be positioned relative to the dental chair?

   a. parallel
   b. 10 degrees
   c. 20 degrees
   d. 30 degrees

4. What disorder or disease would cause the patient to have a loss of postural stability, general stiffness, and a resting tremor of one or both hands?

   a. multiple sclerosis
   b. hypertension
   c. Parkinson's disease
   d. cerebral palsy

5. What disorder or disease' presents with memory loss of recent events, personality changes, and errors in judgment in an aging patient?

   a. ALS
   b. COPD
   c. Alzheimer's disease
   d. seizures

6. Which disorder or disease presents with temporary confusion, staring spells, and uncontrolled jerking movement of arms and legs?

   a. muscular dystrophy
   b. epilepsy
   c. HIV
   d. anemia

7. For what disorder or disease is the acronym FAST used to teach the signs of an impending incident?

    a. CVA

    b. myocardial infarction

    c. anaphylaxis

    d. angina

8. Which disorder or disease is a cancer of the white blood cells and has symptoms of easy bleeding, frequent oral infections, gingival enlargement, and ulcerations?

    a. leukemia

    b. hemophilia

    c. endocarditis

    d. anemia

9. What medication is required after a patient has a joint replacement due to osteoarthritis before dental visits?

    a. corticosteroid

    b. acetaminophen

    c. anti-inflammatory

    d. antibiotic

10. Which disorder or disease presents with a depressive phase and manic phase where the patient may show a lack of interest and concentration and may then become irritable and angry?

    a. panic disorder

    b. schizophrenia

    c. bipolar

    d. intellectual disability

CERTIFICATION REVIEW

1. Which of the following is the best approach for calming an anxious and dissatisfied patient?

    a. Interrupt to explain the situation.

    b. Employ humor to diffuse the anger.

    c. Listen carefully and silently.

    d. Walk away and notify the dentist.

2. What should the role of the dental assistant with special needs patients include?

    a. referring patient questions to business office staff

    b. diagnosing a patient medial emergency

    c. making the patient feel comfortable

    d. prescribing a sedative to the patient

3. What is the best time to schedule a diabetic patient's appointment?

    a. after meal time

    b. in the early morning

    c. before meal time

    d. in the late evening

4. What action should be taken for an older patient experiencing orthostatic hypotension (postural hypotension)?

    a. Administer sublingual nitroglycerin.

    b. Move them from supine to upright position.

    c. Place them in a subsupine position.

    d. Turn them on their left side.

5. What action should be taken for a pregnant patient experiencing pressure on the vena cava during the third trimester?

    a. Reschedule the treatment.
    b. Prepare an ammonia inhalant.
    c. Place patient in a subsupine position.
    d. Turn patient on her left side.

6. Who needs to provide consent for dental treatment of patients with special needs?

    a. patient over 21 years
    b. case manager
    c. physician
    d. legal guardian

7. For which disease or disorder is aspirin use contraindicated due to its blood-thinning properties?

    a. hemophilia
    b. arthritis
    c. diabetes
    d. heart disease

8. What is the best method for the communicator to provide patient education to a hearing-impaired patient?

    a. Speak to the caregiver.
    b. Point to the object and speak loudly.
    c. Write out all directions.
    d. Make eye contact and speak slowly.

9. For which disease or disorder would the patient's medical record indicate that they receive dialysis weekly?

    a. cardiovascular
    b. respiratory
    c. kidney
    d. endocrine

10. Which of the following is one sign of anaphylactic shock?

    a. erythema
    b. itching
    c. respiratory distress
    d. rise in blood pressure

CHAPTER APPLICATION

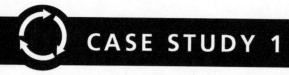

CASE STUDY 1

The first patient with AIDS to be seen in the office is scheduled for an appointment the next day. The dentist calls an office meeting to discuss best practice treatment for the patient.

1. What oral signs may be present with a patient diagnosed with AIDS?

   _____

   _____

   _____

2. Can the dentist refuse to treat the patient with AIDS? Explain.

   _____

   _____

   _____

3. How is AIDS transmitted?

   _____

   _____

   _____

4. What poses a risk of having AIDS transmitted by this patient in the office?

   _____

   _____

   _____

Critical Thinking

Rodriguez is scheduled for a new patient examination. The patient's medical record states that he experienced anxiety during treatment with his previous dentist.

1. How are the signs of anxiety expressed by a patient when they become very anxious?

   _____

   _____

   _____

2. How can the dental team help calm the anxious patient?

   _____

   _____

   _____

CHAPTER 14

Pharmacology

SPECIFIC INSTRUCTIONAL OBJECTIVES

At the completion of this chapter, you will be able to meet these objectives:

1. Use the terms presented in this chapter.
2. State why it is important for the dental assistant to study pharmacology.
3. Discuss the significance of drug laws.
4. Explain the process of new drug development.
5. Recognize that a drug might be known by several names.
6. Identify the drug references available.
7. Discuss how drug dosages are calculated.
8. Compare and contrast the different routes of drug administration.
9. Outline the steps the body uses to process a drug.
10. Identify the information that belongs in each part of a prescription.
11. Provide the English meanings of the common Latin abbreviations used for prescriptions.
12. Discuss the regulations governing prescription drugs.
13. Recognize the signs of a substance use disorder in a dental patient.
14. Define what is meant by a therapeutic action of a drug.
15. Differentiate among the various types of adverse drug reactions.
16. Discuss the types of drugs commonly administered in a dental office.
17. Compare and contrast aspirin, ibuprofen, and acetaminophen.
18. Discuss the dangers of inappropriate use of antibiotics.
19. Discuss the types of drugs commonly prescribed in a dental office.
20. Discuss the drugs that are specific to dental disease.

21. Recognize commonly used dental local anesthetics by name and concentration.

22. Discuss the reasons for selection of a local anesthetic with or without a vasoconstrictor.

23. Recognize medications on the medical history that may impact dental care.

24. Recognize common medications used for the following:

    a. cardiovascular disease

    b. endocrine disorders

    c. psychiatric disorders

    d. neurological disorders

    e. osteoporosis

    f. substance abuse

25. Explain the oral side effects of medications used for:

    a. cardiovascular disease

    b. endocrine disorders

    c. psychiatric disorders

    d. neurological disorders

    e. osteoporosis

    f. cancer chemotherapy

26. Apply treatment modifications for patient management changes for patients taking:

    a. cardiovascular drugs

    b. endocrine drugs

    c. cancer chemotherapy

    d. osteoporosis medications

    e. Antabuse or Methadone

VOCABULARY BUILDER

Matching

Match each term with the appropriate definition.

1. _____ adverse

2. _____ elixir

3. _____ narcotic

4. _____ patent

5. _____ relapse

6. _____ suspension

7. _____ toxic

8. _____ analgesic

9. _____ anabolic

10. _____ vasoconstrictor

a. a sweetened, aromatic solution of alcohol and water

b. the exclusive right granted by a government to an inventor to manufacture, use, or sell an invention for a certain number of years

c. a class of substances that produce stupor or sleep

d. occurrence of effect that is not desired

e. recurrence of symptoms of a disease after a period of recovery

f. poisonous

g. a system consisting of small particles kept dispersed by agitation or by the molecular motion in the surrounding medium

h. building up of body tissues

i. a drug that relieves pain

j. drug causing constriction or narrowing of the blood vessels

Fill in the Blank

Please fill in the blank with one of the choices provided.

decrease   euphoria   symptoms

skin   aromatic   Pharmacology

1. A transdermal patch is an adhesive patch that is applied to the _____.

2. Orthostatic hypotension is a result of a _____ in blood pressure to below normal.

3. A state of intense happiness is known as _____.

CHAPTER REVIEW

Multiple Choice

1. Which of the following is the study of all drugs?

   a. Medicine

   b. Addiction

   c. Pharmacology

   d. Parenteral

2. Patients recovering from substance use disorder related to narcotics may be taking methadone. These patients can be treated for dental pain with an opioid.

   a. Both statements are true.

   b. Both statements are false.

   c. The first statement is true; the second statement is false.

   d. The second statement is true; the first statement is false.

3. Which of the following is correct regarding treatment for cancer?

    a. Patients do not need to have an oral evaluation prior to the start of cancer chemotherapy.

    b. It is not important to correct all sources of potential infection from the oral cavity.

    c. The patient can safely have dental treatment at any time during cancer chemotherapy.

    d. Xerostomia is a common side effect of cancer chemotherapy.

4. Overuse of antibiotics may lead to which of the following?

    a. drowsiness

    b. orthostatic hypotension

    c. greater effect of the antibiotics

    d. bacterial resistance against the drug

5. Which of the following medications can be used to treat candidiasis?

    a. acyclovir

    b. nystatin

    c. penicillin

    d. docosanol

6. Which of the following is not a potential adverse effect of aspirin?

    a. reduced clotting ability of blood

    b. drowsiness

    c. stomach irritability

    d. allergic reaction

7. Which of the following is the most common sedative used in the dental office?

    a. barbiturates

    b. benzodiazepines

    c. chloral hydrate

    d. amide local anesthetics

8. A patient is given a medication for high blood pressure and experiences a severe drop in blood pressure. This type of adverse drug reaction is known as what type of reaction?

    a. side effect

    b. Type I allergic

    c. Type II allergic

    d. toxic reaction

9. Which of the following drug schedules cannot be phones into the pharmacy and must have a written prescription?

    a. Schedule I

    b. Schedule II

    c. Schedule III

    d. Schedule IV

10. Most drugs are excreted by the

    a. liver.

    b. kidneys.

    c. lungs.

    d. heart.

Matching

Match the local anesthetic with the correct concentration of anesthetic agent and vasoconstrictor (epinephrine).

1. _____ lidocaine

2. _____ mepivacaine

3. _____ prilocaine

4. _____ bupivacaine

5. _____ articaine

a. 3%, no vasoconstrictor

b. 2%, 1:100,000

c. 4%, 1:100,000

d. .5%, 1:200,000

e. 4%, no vasoconstrictor

Match the local anesthetic with the correct brand name.

1. _____ lidocaine
2. _____ mepivacaine
3. _____ prilocaine
4. _____ bupivacaine
5. _____ articaine

a. Marcaine
b. Septocaine
c. Octocaine
d. Carbocaine
e. Citanest

CERTIFICATION REVIEW

Multiple Choice

1. A patient who is taking an angiotensin-converting enzyme would likely have which condition?

   a. diabetes
   b. epilepsy
   c. angina
   d. hypertension

2. For which pregnancy category has testing in pregnant animals showed harm to fetus, and/or there are no available studies in animals or humans?

   a. A
   b. B
   c. C
   d. D

3. Valium (diazepam) is considered which DEA schedule?

   a. I
   b. II
   c. III
   d. IV

4. What is the brand name for codeine and acetaminophen?

   a. Percocet
   b. Tylenol #3
   c. Demerol
   d. Vicodin

5. What is the antibiotic prophylactically regimen for a patient who is able to take oral medication with no medication allergies?

   a. amoxicillin, 2 g
   b. amoxicillin, 500 mg
   c. clindamycin, 500 mg
   d. clindamycin, 600 mg

6. Nitroglycerin is considered a

   a. vasoconstrictor.
   b. vasodilator.
   c. anticoagulant.
   d. diuretic.

7. The drug of choice for a yeast infection is

   a. Nystatin.
   b. Abreva.
   c. Nitrostat.
   d. Plavix.

8. Which of the following is true regarding antibiotics?

   a. They are effective against viral infections.

   b. They do not have many common side effects.

   c. Overuse could lead to the formation of a resistant strain.

   d. They only kill the bad bacteria.

9. Which of the following conditions requires an antibiotic prophylactic?

   a. heart murmur

   b. congenital heart disease

   c. history of bypass surgery

   d. mitral valve prolapse

10. If antibiotic prophylactic is necessary, which of the following procedures would require the patient take them?

   a. radiographs

   b. fluoride treatment

   c. sealants

   d. periodontal probing

CHAPTER APPLICATION

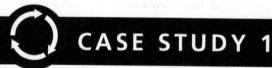

CASE STUDY 1

Gail arrives at the dental office and is scheduled for a recare appointment. When the dental assistant updates Gail's medical history, she notices she is taking a new medication, Fosamax (alendronate).

1. What class of medications is Fosamax?

   _____

   _____

2. What condition is Gail most likely taking Fosamax for?

   _____

   _____

3. What is a rare but serious condition that can occur if taking Fosamax and trauma is caused to the jaw?

   _____

   _____

Critical Thinking

The physician provides directions to the pharmacist within the body of the prescription. The directions include abbreviations of the name and strength of the drug dose. This information is often in the form of a Latin abbreviation. Define the following Latin abbreviations.

1. disp

_____

_____

2. qid

_____

_____

3. qh

_____

_____

4. q4h

_____

_____

5. PO

_____

_____

CHAPTER 15

Medical Emergencies

SPECIFIC INSTRUCTIONAL OBJECTIVES

At the completion of this chapter, you will be able to meet these objectives:

1. Use the terms provided in this chapter.
2. Discuss prevention of a medical emergency through collection of an accurate patient history.
3. Recognize signs of an anxious or fearful patient.
4. Discuss ASA classifications of Medical Risk.
5. Explain prevention of a medical emergency through staff preparation.
6. Explain prevention of a medical emergency through office preparation.
7. Compare and contrast the management of postural hypotension and vasovagal syncope.
8. Compare and contrast the signs and symptoms of postural hypotension and vasovagal syncope.
9. Identify the predisposing factors to postural hypotension.
10. Compare and contrast the signs and symptoms of asthma and hyperventilation.
11. Compare and contrast the management of asthma and hyperventilation.
12. Discuss the management of chronic obstructive pulmonary disease.
13. Define adrenal disorders.
14. Discuss the management of an acute adrenal crisis in the dental office.
15. Describe the anatomical structure of the thyroid gland.
16. Compare and contrast hypothyroidism and hyperthyroidism.
17. Describe the protocol in managing a thyroid related medical emergency in the dental office.
18. Differentiate between type I, type II, prediabetes, and gestational diabetes.
19. Discuss the complications of diabetes.

20. List the steps in managing a diabetic emergency in the dental office.
21. Compare and contrast angina and myocardial infarction.
22. Discuss the management of an angina attack in the dental office.
23. Discuss the management of a myocardial infarction in the dental office.
24. Define cardiac arrest.
25. Define congestive heart failure.
26. Discuss the protocol for managing acute pulmonary edema in the dental office.
27. Differentiate between epilepsy and seizures.
28. Discuss generalized seizures.
29. Outline the steps in the management of a seizure in the dental office.
30. Differentiate between an ischemic cerebrovascular accident and a hemorrhagic cerebrovascular accident.
31. Outline the steps in the management of a cerebrovascular accident in the dental office.
32. Identify common dental allergens.
33. Outline the steps in the management of an allergic reaction in the dental office.
34. State the protocol for managing an airway obstruction in the conscious patient.
35. State the role of the dental assistant in managing a medical emergency.

VOCABULARY BUILDER

Matching

Match each term with the appropriate definition.

1. _____ antigen

2. _____ chronic

3. _____ diastolic

4. _____ embolus

5. _____ euthroid

6. _____ systolic

7. _____ polyp

8. _____ thrombus

9. _____ retinopathy

10. _____ phagocytes

a. normal thyroid function

b. disease of the retina of the eye that may lead to blindness

c. blood clot in a vessel that leads to occlusion

d. blood clot that detaches and travels from a larger vessel to a smaller one, resulting in occlusion of the smaller vessel

e. substances that stimulate the production of antibodies

f. contraction of the heart, particularly the ventricles

g. long term as in a disease

h. cell that engulfs and destroys invaders such as bacteria and viruses

i. post-systolic relaxation of the heart, particularly referring to the ventricles

j. growth protruding from a mucous membrane

Fill in the Blank

Please fill in the blank with one of the choices provided.

hypovolemia	diabetes	nephropathy
tachycardia	urination	Blood

1. Nocturia is frequent _____ at night

2. A low volume of circulating blood in the body is known as _____.

CHAPTER REVIEW

True or False

1. Blood pressure is recorded using a sphygmomanometer and a stethoscope.

   a. Both statements are true.

   b. Both statements are false.

   c. The first statement is true; the second statement is false.

   d. The first statement is false; the second statement is true.

2. When taking blood pressure, the upper number is the systolic blood pressure and the lower number is the diastolic blood pressure.

   a. Both statements are true.

   b. Both statements are false.

   c. The first statement is true; the second statement is false

   d. The first statement is false; the second statement is true.

3. A normal adult pulse rate ranges from 80 to 120 beats per minute. A pulse that is fast may be a sign of tachycardia.

   a. Both statements are true.

   b. Both statements are false.

   c. The first statement is true; the second statement is false.

   d. The first statement is false; the second statement is true.

4. Syncope is one of the most common medical emergencies that occurs in the dental office. If the patient experiences an episode of vasodepressor syncope, it is important to keep the patient in an upright position.

   a. Both statements are true.

   b. Both statements are false.

   c. The first statement is true; the second statement is false.

   d. The first statement is false; the second statement is true.

5. The systolic blood pressure is the upper number and is the pressure when the left ventricle is pumping the blood to the remaining vessels in the body. The diastolic blood pressure is the lower number and is when the heart is at rest and is refilling with blood.

   a. Both statements are true.

   b. Both statements are false.

   c. The first statement is true; the second statement is false

   d. The first statement is false; the second statement is true.

6. Managing the patient with a history of postural hypotension includes obtaining an accurate medical history. As a preventive measure, the dental chair should be raised quickly from supine to upright at the end of the appointment so the patient can adjust to the change in position.

   a. Both statements are true.
   b. Both statements are false.
   c. The first statement is true; the second statement is false.
   d. The first statement is false; the second statement is true.

7. Myxedema coma is an acute emergency related to hyperthyroidism. Myxedema coma is managed in the hospital by administration of large amounts of electrolytes as well as T3 and T4.

   a. Both statements are true.
   b. Both statements are false.
   c. The first statement is true; the second statement is false.
   d. The first statement is false; the second statement is true.

8. The chronic complications of diabetes include damage to small and large blood vessels. The chronic complications of diabetes are mostly seen in the Type II diabetic.

   a. Both statements are true.
   b. Both statements are false.
   c. The first statement is true; the second statement is false.
   d. The first statement is false; the second statement is true.

Multiple Choice

1. Which of the following are ways that the dental assistant can help in preventing and managing a medical emergency in the dental office?

   a. reviewing the medical history with every new patient
   b. reviewing and updating the medical history with every returning patient
   c. completing BLS and CPR refresher classes to maintain updated credentials
   d. participating in dental office practice drills
   e. all of the above

2. During dental treatment, a patient suddenly gives the universal sign of choking. The patient is conscious. Upon immediate termination of treatment, what should the dental professional do?

   a. Perform the Heimlich maneuver.
   b. There is no need to do anything.
   c. Allow the patient to cough so the object can be dislodged.
   d. Look to see if you can visualize the object.

3. Which of the following statements is correct regarding the signs and symptoms of hyperventilation?

   a. Hyperventilation is characterized by constriction of the bronchioles.
   b. Patients who suffer from hyperventilation exhibit a wheezing sound on exhalation.
   c. Hyperventilation is triggered by an allergen.
   d. Numbness of the extremities and perioral areas may occur during hyperventilation.

4. Which of the following is part of the management protocol for asthma?

   a. Request patient to place cupped hands over the nose and mouth and breathe.

   b. Administer a bronchodilator.

   c. Place the patient in the supine position.

   d. Administer Valium.

5. Which of the following is a chronic complication of diabetes that can lead to a loss of sensation in the feet?

a. neuropathy

b. nephropathy

c. retinopathy

d. microangiopathy

Matching

Match the type of diabetes with the correct description.

Term

1. _____ Type I diabetes

2. _____ Type II diabetes

3. _____ Gestational diabetes

4. _____ Prediabetes

Description

a. occurs during pregnancy

b. destruction of beta cells of pancreas result in lack of insulin production

c. linked to obesity

d. glucose levels elevated but not high enough for a diagnosis of diabetes

Match the term with its description.

Term

5. _____ cerebral infarction

6. _____ cerebral embolism

7. _____ cerebral hemorrhage

8. _____ hemiplegia

9. _____ transient ischemic attacks

Description

a. rupture of a blood vessel

b. weakness, numbness, or paralysis on one side

c. blood clot

d. stroke-like symptoms that disappear in 24 hours

e. sudden onset caused by blood loss to brain

CERTIFICATION REVIEW

1. The most common and least life-threatening emergency that may occur in the dental office is

a. allergic reaction.

b. anaphylactic shock.

c. syncope.

d. angina pectoris.

2. In the dental office, a vasodepressor syncope occurred. This incident is also known as

a. allergic reaction.

b. anaphylactic shock.

c. fainting.

d. seizure.

3. The wheezing and breathlessness of an asthma patient are due to the narrowing of small airways called

a. the trachea.

b. the nasal cavity.

c. bronchioles.

d. lungs.

4. Which of the following is a severe, life-threatening allergic reaction?

    a. hyperventilation
    b. hypoglycemia
    c. anaphylactic shock
    d. congestive heart failure

5. Which of the following results from the loss of carbon dioxide from the blood, causing alkalosis?

    a. hyperglycemia
    b. hyperventilation
    c. hypoglycemia
    d. hemiplegia

6. Which type of diabetes has a genetic component that results in a destruction of the beta cells of the pancreas that produce insulin and occurs between the ages of 10 and 16?

    a. Type I
    b. Type II
    c. epilepsy
    d. hypoglycemia

7. This is the result of the pancreas not producing sufficient insulin.

    a. a seizure
    b. hyperventilation
    c. diabetes
    d. angina

8. Which medical emergency is sublingual nitroglycerin is administered for?

    a. syncope
    b. angina attack
    c. asthma attack
    d. hyperglycemia

9. A diabetic patient's appointment time is best scheduled

    a. in the morning after meal time.
    b. before meal time.
    c. in the late evening.
    d. in the afternoon.

10. Which of the following is a sign of anaphylactic shock?

    a. chest pain
    b. urticaria
    c. respiratory distress
    d. rise in blood pressure

CHAPTER APPLICATION

 CASE STUDY 1

The 9 a.m. patient arrives to the dental office and realizes that she forgot to take her premedication antibiotics. She has no history of allergic reactions and is given four tablets of 500 milligrams of amoxicillin in the dental office. The patient is asked to wait in the treatment room prior to the start of treatment. While you are speaking with the patient, you notice a red rash on the patient's face. The rash was not present when the patient came to the office. The patient also states that her face feels hot. The rash does not seem to be progressing, and the patient is able to breathe without any problems. You immediately summon the dentist.

1. What could you suspect the patient experiencing?

   _____

2. Based on your response to the question above, what is the appropriate medication to give to the patient?

   _____

 CASE STUDY 2

Kelsey arrives for her four unit bridge appointment. Everything goes well for the appointment, and the doctor has just finished preparing the teeth. When you raise Kelsey to take the impressions, she suddenly loses consciousness.

3. What do you suspect happened to Kelsey?

   _____

   _____

4. What causes the above condition?

   _____

   _____

5. What are some predisposing factors of this condition?

   _____

   _____

6. What is the protocol for prevention of the above condition?

   _____

   _____

   _____

   _____

Prevention and Nutrition

CHAPTER 16

Oral Health and Preventive Techniques

SPECIFIC INSTRUCTIONAL OBJECTIVES

At the completion of this chapter, you will be able to meet these objectives:

1. Use terms presented in this chapter.
2. Explain how biofilm affects the tooth, gingiva, and periodontium.
3. Describe strategies that are part of a good prevention plan.
4. Identify oral hygiene tips that will aid each age group.
5. Order activities for good oral self-care practice.
6. Provide guidance in selection of the ideal toothbrush.
7. Explain special considerations for the use of a toothbrush.
8. Demonstrate toothbrushing techniques.
9. Describe the purpose of the ingredients contained within most dentifrices.
10. Recommend different types of dental floss based on oral findings.
11. Demonstrate proper dental flossing.
12. Evaluate oral self-care using disclosing agents and biofilm indices.
13. Compare oral hygiene aids and their uses.
14. Describe fluoride and its use in good self-care.
15. Discuss benefits and mechanism of systemic and topical fluoride.
16. Select oral hygiene aids for patients with prosthetic appliances.
17. Compare the design of products to assist patients with disabilities to perform oral self-care effectively.
18. Describe the mission of dental public health.

VOCABULARY BUILDER

Matching

Match each term with the appropriate definition.

1. _____ xero-
2. _____ stom
3. _____ -ia
4. _____ sol

a. condition
b. mouth or mouth-like
c. dry
d. liquid

5. _____ phylaxis
6. _____ alba
7. _____ mal-
8. _____ inflame

a. white matter
b. cause redness and heat
c. bad
d. process of guarding

9. _____ pellicle
10. _____ calculus
11. _____ dentifrice
12. _____ materia alba

a. toothpaste
b. thin, clear film of protein on surface of teeth
c. accumulation of food debris and microorganisms around gumline
d. hard, calcified deposits of mineralized biofilm

13. _____ fluorapatite
14. _____ hydroxyapatite
15. _____ ingest
16. _____ index

a. mineral formed from in presence of fluoride; hardens teeth
b. number indicating a relationship
c. mineral storage form for calcium and phosphorus
d. consume something orally

Fill in the Blank

recession   periodontal pocket   hygiene

systemic   suppuration   fluorapatite

1. The diseased space between the gingiva and the surface of the tooth is called a _____.

2. _____ is the withdrawal of the gingival tissue from the tooth.

3. The dental assistant records the presence of _____ upon noticing pus forming in the sulcus.

4. The patient obtains _____ fluoride by ingesting fluoride rich food and fluoridated water.

CHAPTER REVIEW

True or False

Circle whether the answer is true or false.

1. **T F** When developing personal oral hygiene goals for patients, each patient should be treated as an individual.

2. **T F** Topical fluoride can assist in the remineralization of decalcified areas.

3. **T F** There is only one recommended method to properly remove biofilm buildup on teeth.

4. **T F** In order to protect users from the condition of fluoride toxicity, dentifrice should not contain fluoride.

5. **T F** The ADA awards a Seal of Acceptance classification to products that are safe and effective for self-care.

6. All of these statements about denture care is true EXCEPT

   a. dentures should be removed every night.

   b. dentures should be stored in water.

   c. the basin used to clean denture is lined with a towel and filled with water.

   d. after receiving a denture, the need for dental care is over.

Multiple Choice

1. How soon after brushing their teeth may a patient expect biofilm to begin forming?

   a. within in seconds

   b. 2 hours

   c. 4 to 6 hours

   d. 12 hours

2. A condition where the enamel shows varying degrees of white areas beneath biofilm could be due to

   a. demineralization.

   b. enamel hyperplasia.

   c. excessive brushing.

   d. xerostomia.

3. What can be placed over faulty unions of enamel in newly erupted teeth to help prevent caries?

   a. amalgam

   b. disclosing solution

   c. cement

   d. sealants

4. At what age should emphasis be placed on nutrition and the patient's concern about peer pressure and bad breath?

   a. 5–8 years

   b. 9–12 years

   c. 13–15 years

   d. 16–19 years

5. How many tooth surfaces are cleaned using a toothbrush?

   a. 2

   b. 3

   c. 4

   d. 5

6. How many tooth surfaces are cleaned when flossing?

   a. 2

   b. 3

   c. 4

   d. 5

7. What is the most important criteria in selecting a toothbrush for a patient?

    a. It has nylon bristles.

    b. It is the patient's favorite type of brush.

    c. It is the correct size and shape for the patient's mouth.

    d. It has the highest ADA rating.

8. What is the systematic sequence recommended for brushing teeth so no areas are missed?

    a. Always start in the upper right and end on the lower right.

    b. Start at the midline to the posterior of each quadrant.

    c. Brush occlusal surfaces first.

    d. Start and end in the same place.

9. What can be suggested to ensure coverage of every surface when brushing teeth?

    a. Brush all facial surfaces first.

    b. Brush all surfaces of one tooth at a time.

    c. Overlap the previous stroke with each brush placement.

    d. Clean one quadrant at a time.

10. How many times and for how long should be recommended to the patient when brushing their teeth?

    a. 2 times for 2 minutes

    b. 3 times for 3 minutes

    c. 4 times for 2 minutes

    d. 4 times for 3 minutes

11. Which brushing technique has the bristles gently pressed into the interproximal area while using a back-and-forth vibratory stroke?

    a. Bass

    b. Fones

    c. Stillman

    d. Charters

    e. roll

12. Which brushing technique is being used when the patient closes their teeth together, holds the brush at a 90-degree angle, and moves the brush in a circular motion over both the maxillary and mandibular teeth?

    a. Bass

    b. Fones

    c. Stillman

    d. Charters

    e. roll

13. Which brushing technique is being used when the patient closes their teeth together, holds the brush at a 90-degree angle, and moves the brush in a back-and-forth motion over both the maxillary and mandibular teeth?

    a. Bass

    b. modified Bass

    c. scrub

    d. Charters

    e. roll

14. The patient is instructed to place the brush against the attached gingiva at a 45-degree angle and slowly move the brush toward the occlusal in a vertical motion. What brushing technique is being used?

    a. Bass

    b. modified Bass

    c. Stillman

    d. Charters

    e. roll

15. Which brushing technique has the bristles pointed at a 45-degree angle into the sulcus while using a gentle, short vibrating motion followed by a vertical motion toward the occlusal surface?

    a. Bass

    b. modified Bass

    c. scrub

    d. Charters

    e. roll

16. Why is it important for each family member have their own toothpaste tube?

    a. each member's need for a different type of toothpaste

    b. cross-contamination of the tube

    c. preference for different flavors

    d. different cosmetic desires

17. From what surfaces does floss best remove biofilm?

    a. occlusal

    b. facial and buccal

    c. interproximal

    d. all surfaces

18. When dispensing dental floss, an appropriate length is about _____ inches.

    a. 4

    b. 10

    c. 18

    d. 25

19. Which type of floss enable the floss to slide more easily between tight contacts of the teeth?

    a. unwaxed

    b. waxed

    c. monofilament

    d. flavored

20. The floss is gently wrapped around the _____ fingers of each hand to stabilize while flossing.

    a. index

    b. middle

    c. fourth

    d. little

21. How much floss should be held be the two index fingers while placing the floss between the teeth?

    a. 1–2 inches

    b. 2–3 inches

    c. 3–4 inches

    d. 4–6 inches

22. How can the use of dental floss harm the gingival tissue?

    a. snapping the floss through the contacts

    b. forcing the floss into the gingiva

    c. placing floss too far under the gumline

    d. all of these

23. What should be done when disclosing if a patient has tooth-colored restorations or crowns to avoid staining?

    a. It is not recommended to disclose.

    b. Place fluoride over the areas.

    c. Apply lubricant to teeth first.

    d. Use nonstaining agents.

24. What aid can be added to the patient's self-care to floss into closed contacts?

    a. floss holder

    b. floss threader

    c. gauze strip

    d. interdental brush

CERTIFICATION REVIEW

1. What is recorded when the patient's teeth exhibit mottling and pitting on the enamel surface resulting from excessive fluoride?

    a. systemic fluoride

    b. fluoride toxicity

    c. fluoride poisoning

    d. fluorosis

2. For which condition would mouthwashes and sprays be added to the patient's hygiene routine to promote their salivary flow?

    a. dental caries

    b. candidiasis

    c. gingivitis

    d. xerostomia

3. Why is it an advantage to add dental sealants to the preventive program?

    a. eliminates the need for brushing

    b. prevents early childhood caries syndrome

    c. prevents dental fluorosis

    d. protects enamel from biofilm and acids

4. What may occur if the patient brushes vigorously?

    a. bone loss

    b. enamel abrasion

    c. gingivitis

    d. mottled enamel

5. What can be recommended to help the patient identify the presence of biofilm?

    a. dentifrice

    b. xylitol

    c. disclosing agent

    d. mouthwash

6. What sweetener is in some chewing gum that may be recommended because it inhibits colonization of biofilm and has been shown to prevent caries?

    a. sucrose

    b. xylitol

    c. agave

    d. stevia

7. The patient is consistently missing the biofilm below the gumline. What is the most commonly recommended toothbrushing method?

    a. Bass

    b. Stillman

    c. Charter

    d. Fones

8. What brushing technique is being used when a patient uses short back-and-forth vibratory strokes with the bristles directed apically and placed on the gingiva and cervical area of the tooth?

    a. Bass

    b. modified Bass

    c. Stillman

    d. Charters

    e. roll

9. What mineral nutrient enhances remineralization of the tooth and causes a significant reduction in dental caries?

   a. phosphorus
   b. calcium
   c. iron
   d. fluoride

10. What is the single most common chronic disease of childhood?

    a. diabetes
    b. cancer
    c. obesity
    d. tooth decay

CHAPTER APPLICATION

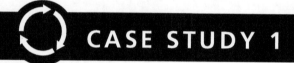

CASE STUDY 1

Daniel is 10 years old and is new to the city and to the dental office. Upon examination, the dentist notices white and pitted spots on all of the permanent anterior teeth. The dentist asks the mother, "What is Daniel's source of fluoride?"

The mother explains, "I give Daniel dietary fluoride supplements because we lived in the country and used well water. Our previous dentist tested the water and there was no fluoride present."

Dentist: "Have you had your current water tested?"

Mother: "I have not."

Dentist: "I would like you to have your water tested. I believe these white and pitted spots may be cause by the fluoride. After the water is tested, please call the office and tell me the results of the test."

1. How does a patient receive fluoride systemically?

   _____

   _____

   _____

2. What may occur if all systemic forms of fluoride are not considered prior to ingestion?

   _____

   _____

CASE STUDY 2

Claire, age 42, recently acquired dental coverage from her employer and is registering as a first-time dental patient. The dentist has completed her oral health diagnosis and found areas of biofilm primarily at the gumline and in most interproximal areas, gingivitis, and the beginning stages of periodontitis. Dental charting shows some restorations. Patient x-rays indicate that demineralization is also occurring in certain areas.

1. What steps are recommended to motivate this patient to better oral health?

_____

2. What type of oral health home care should be emphasized?

_____

Critical Thinking

1. The dental assistant is requested to take the biofilm score for a 12-year-old patient. All permanent teeth through the second molars are present. After disclosing, the assistant records 14 surfaces with biofilm present. What is the biofilm score?

_____

_____

_____

_____

CHAPTER 17

Nutrition

SPECIFIC INSTRUCTIONAL OBJECTIVES

At the completion of this chapter, you will be able to meet these objectives:

1. Use terms presented in this chapter.
2. Describe the role of nutrition in the health of the human body and oral development.
3. Discuss the six classes of nutrients and their functions and sources.
4. Identify the food groups and their nutrients.
5. Discuss calories, metabolic rate, and BMR.
6. Interpret food labels.
7. Summarize food safety issues.
8. Compare governmental dietary recommendations.
9. Explain the feature of MyPlate in selecting food groups.
10. Explain the role of nutrition upon dental caries, gingivitis and periodontal disease.
11. Describe the role of carbohydrates in the diet and its effect on the teeth.
12. Discuss the relationship between nutrition and systemic disease.
13. Explain the special dietary needs of patients in specific dental situations.
14. Describe religious and cultural considerations regarding diet.
15. Discuss the implications of eating disorders
16. Discuss the dental assistant's role in nutrition.

VOCABULARY BUILDER

Matching

Match each term with the appropriate definition.

1. _____ -lysis

2. _____ gluc

3. _____ -ose

4. _____ -osis

5. _____ plast

6. _____ somni-

7. _____ lact

8. _____ amylase

9. _____ dialysis

10. _____ electrolyte

11. _____ halitosis

12. _____ insomnia

13. _____ nutrition

a. condition

b. sleep

c. milk

d. sugar

e. forms names of sugars

f. growth

g. breaking down

a. process of using food for growth

b. regulates electric charge and flow of water

c. enzyme that converts starch/glycogen into simple sugar

d. removes uric acid from blood

e. sleeplessness

f. breath

Fill in the Blank

Please fill in the blank with one of the choices provided.

diuretic

fermentable

Calorie

BMI

metabolic

Collagen

glycogen

energy

1. _____ is the measurement of fat and muscle mass.

2. The amount of energy from food required to raise 1 kilogram of water 1 degree Celsius is a(an) _____.

3. A food capable of producing dental decay is _____.

4 _____ is a fibrous protein found in bone, cartilage, skin and connective tissue.

5. A substance that increases the volume of urine is a _____.

6. Yeasts and molds that can cause a chemical reaction that splits compounds into simple substances are _____.

7. A _____ chemical process produces energy needed for life.

CHAPTER REVIEW

Matching

Match the vitamin with how the body uses it.

Vitamin

1. _____ vitamin A
2. _____ vitamin D
3. _____ vitamin K
4. _____ vitamin C
5. _____ vitamin B1

Use

a. promotes blood clotting and coagulation
b. gives strength to epithelial tissue
c. acts to hold cells together
d. promotes tooth development
e. promotes nerve function

Match the mineral with how the body uses it.

Mineral

1. _____ calcium
2. _____ magnesium
3. _____ potassium
4. _____ sodium
5. _____ zinc

Use

a. promotes immune system function
b. promotes kidney, heart, digestive, and nerve function
c. maintains strong bones and teeth
d. maintains balance of body fluids
e. supports contraction/relaxation of muscles

Match the nutritional deficiency with the oral impact.

Nutritional Deficiency

1. _____ calcium
2. _____ magnesium
3. _____ fluoride
4. _____ vitamin A
5. _____ vitamin C

Oral Impact

a. increased caries susceptibility
b. dark red, inflamed gingiva
c. generalized gingivitis
d. underdeveloped enamel
e. poor mineralization of the tooth

True or False

Circle whether the answer is true or false.

1. **T** **F** Nutrients are everything that is ingested via the mouth.

2. **T** **F** All vitamins fall in one of two groups: water soluble or fat soluble.

3. **T** **F** Water is the most abundant nutrient in the body.

4. **T** **F** One of the leading causes of death of Americans over age 40 is heart disease, and a contributing factor may be the consumption of too many fats.

5. **T** **F** Care should be taken when eating fats and lipids because these foods are typically cariogenic.

6. **T   F**   Water soluble nutrients are stored in the body and not destroyed by cooking.

7. **T   F**   People can eat large amounts of food yet still be undernourished, that is, lacking the correct nutrients for the body.

8. **T   F**   The percent daily value on food labels is based on 2000 calories.

9. **T   F**   When the food label indicates that the food is organic, it must have been grown without herbicides, chemical pesticides, or fertilizers.

10. **T   F**   Iron deficiency may result in anemia.

Multiple Choice

1. All of these describe the relationship between water and salivary gland function EXCEPT

   a. the gland will not develop without water.

   b. saliva quality is dependent on water intake.

   c. dehydration may occur with decreased water intake.

   d. protective effects for the mouth are lessened.

2. The major minerals are calcium, phosphorus, potassium, sodium, chlorine, magnesium, and

   a. copper.

   b. sulfur.

   c. chromium.

   d. manganese.

3. Which nutrient(s) are found in fruits, grains, legumes, and some vegetable roots?

   a. proteins

   b. fats

   c. carbohydrates

   d. vitamin C

4. Which nutrient is so vital that the body can only survive 3 days without it?

   a. fats

   b. proteins

   c. carbohydrates

   d. water

5. Which food group provides vitamins A, C, and E and folic acid?

   a. fruits

   b. vegetables

   c. proteins

   d. grains

6. All foods from meat, poultry, seafood, beans, and eggs are a part of the _____ group.

   a. protein

   b. grains

   c. dairy

   d. fruits

7. What should be completed before eating fruits and vegetables?

   a. Peel them.

   b. Soak them in soapy water.

   c. Wash and rinse them.

   d. Refrigerate them.

8. Which snack foods have the highest potential for cariogenic activity?

   a. soft drinks and potato chips

   b. peanut butter and jelly sandwich

   c. fresh fruit and cheese

   d. peanuts and popcorn

9. Which eating disorder is related to an extreme fear of being fat with a distorted body image?

   a. anorexia nervosa

   b. bulimia

   c. pica

   d. chronic dieting syndrome

10. When the assistant compares the patient's diet to the recommended number of servings per day, they are completing _____.

   a. diet modification

   b. a diet diary

   c. the dietary analysis

   d. a food frequency questionnaire

CERTIFICATION REVIEW

1. Which are considered cariogenic?

   a. triglycerides

   b. fat soluble vitamins

   c. refined carbohydrates

   d. proteins

2. Which is a part of a healthy diet to help avoid decay?

   a. whole grains and milk

   b. raw fruits and vegetables

   c. slow-dissolving candies

   d. sticky and salted food

3. Which of the following vitamins is vital for tooth development?

   a. A

   b. E

   c. K

   d. D

4. Which eating disorder presents with erosion on the lingual surfaces of the teeth?

   a. anorexia nervosa

   b. bulimia

   c. female athlete triad

   d. chronic dieting syndrome

5. Why is optimal nutrition important for oral structures during pregnancy?

   a. Permanent teeth are calcified.

   b. Development of the jaws may be affected.

   c. Primary teeth are erupting.

   d. Nutrition does not affect oral structures during pregnancy.

6. Fats (lipids) in normal diets occur in plant and animal foods and are identified as

   a. amino acids.

   b. proteins.

   c. triglycerides.

   d. thiamin.

7. Which food group is highest in sugar?

   a. fruits

   b. vegetables

   c. proteins

   d. grains

8. Which emphasizes balancing healthy eating with exercise?

   a. Dietary Guidelines for Americans

   b. MyPlate

   c. food labels

   d. Food and Drug Administration

9. Which disorder is related to carbohydrate metabolism?

   a. phenylketonuria (PKU)

   b. diabetes

   c. kwashiorkor

   d. osteoporosis

10. What diet modifications are recommended for patients after the first few days after oral surgery?

   a. high-carbohydrate liquid

   b. high-protein liquid

   c. semisoft foods

   d. no modifications

CHAPTER APPLICATION

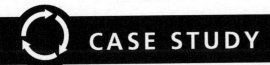

CASE STUDY

Muriel is a 12-year-old patient who has recently had orthodontic appliances delivered. On a routine dental visit, Muriel's oral exam revealed several tissue indications of change since her last visit. These conditions included gingivitis, tissue irritation and swelling, and beginning areas of decalcification. While discussing these conditions with the dental team, Muriel informs them that she has had problems with her appliances breaking and that each time after an adjustment that her mouth is very tender.

1. What vitamin may be deficient and impacting the gingival condition?

2. What information can the assistant discuss regarding the beginning of areas of decalcification?

3. What suggestions can the assistant provide the patient to prevent breaking her appliances?

_____

_____

4. What recommendations can the assistant discuss about her tenderness after adjustment?

_____

_____

X Critical Thinking

Andre is a 16-year-old patient who has had a history of dental caries at each visit. His biofilm record has been average and is improving. The dentist has requested that the dental assistant analyze Andre's 24 hour food diet using the ChooseMyPlate as a guide for the diet analysis and counseling with him.

Andre's 24 hour food survey

Breakfast	orange juice, toast with butter and jelly
Lunch	hamburger, French fries, and soda pop
Snack	small bag of potato chips and soda pop
Dinner	spaghetti, garlic bread and milk
Snack	cookies

1. What food groups are deficient in Andre's diet? Analyze each meal.

Breakfast	orange juice, toast with butter and jelly _____
Lunch	hamburger and bun, French fries, and soda pop _____
Dinner	spaghetti, garlic bread and milk _____

2. What foods in his survey are cariogenic?

_____

_____

_____

3. What recommendation could be made to improve Andre's nutrition and lower his cariogenic foods?

_____

_____

_____

4. What food group is missing the most from Andre's diet?

_____

_____

_____

Assist with Diagnosis and Prevention

The Dental Office

SPECIFIC INSTRUCTIONAL OBJECTIVES

At the completion of this chapter, you will be able to meet these objectives:

1. Use terms presented in this chapter.
2. Describe the design of a dental office, explaining the purpose of each area.
3. Follow safety rules in operating dental equipment.
4. Describe appearance and function of the equipment in the treatment room.
5. Select the best method to sanitize and disinfect equipment.
6. Describe the daily routine to open and close the dental office.
7. Prepare the treatment room for patient seating.
8. Greet and escort the patient to the treatment room.
9. Seat the patient.
10. Dismiss the patient.
11. Assist patients requiring seating accommodations.

VOCABULARY BUILDER

Matching

Match each term with the appropriate definition.

1. _____ –ic
2. _____ con-
3. _____ –ate
4. _____ -able
5. _____ -tory
6. _____ expend
7. _____ cephalo-

a. to put out
b. place equipped for work
c. fit for
d. possessing
e. relating to
f. with
g. head

8. _____ operative	a. body position
9. _____ operatory	b. observation of signs
10. _____ rheostat	c. treatment requiring dental procedures
11. _____ posture	d. regulates electricity to run equipment
12. _____ subsupine	e. lying with head lower than body
13. _____ turbine	f. room dental team performs tasks for patient
14. _____ clinical	g. part in handpiece the produces power

Fill in the Blank

Please fill in the blank with one of the choices provided.

intrusive	expendable	clinic
handpiece	postural hypotension	ergonomics

1. A(an) _____ is an item designed for single use.

2. The layperson's term for _____ is dental drill.

3. The place where outpatients are treated is the _____.

4. Modifying one's method of work to prevent strain injuries is _____.

5. A situation is _____ when it becomes irritating and disturbing.

6. _____ occurs when there is a sudden drop in blood pressure resulting from a change in body position.

CHAPTER REVIEW

True or False

Circle whether the answer is true or false.

1. **T   F**   The sterilization area of the dental office should be near the treatment room.

2. **T   F**   Dental treatment rooms are also called operatories.

3. **T   F**   A reclined position with the patient's head lower than their feet may be called a supine position.

4. **T   F**   The air/water syringe is used to remove saliva and fluids from the patient's mouth.

5. Dental staff cannot wear uniforms outside of work. If protective clothing is not provided, OSHA regulations state that the employer is responsible for laundering or laundry service.

   a. Both statements are true.
   b. Both statements are false.
   c. The first statement is true; the second statement is false.
   d. The first statement is false; the second statement is true.

Matching

Match the room to an office by its design and function.

Room

1. _____ reception desk

2. _____ business office

3. _____ sterilizing area

4. _____ x-ray processing room

Function

a. Near treatment room, has good air circulation to protect from the chemical fumes that may be exhausted.

b. Small room near the treatment rooms. Equipment includes a manual processing tank, drying racks, and a safelight.

c. Area or space where patients can pay bills and schedule appointments. This area may also be used for private conversations with patients.

d. Adjacent to the reception area. Greeting area for the patient and place where telephone calls are received.

Multiple Choice

1. The assistant should arrive early to open the office and prepare for the day's schedule. Which of the following is NOT a part of opening the office?

   a. Turn on the master switches, lights, dental units, vacuum system, and air compressor.
   b. Turn off the water supply to the manual processing tanks.
   c. Change into appropriate clinical clothing and follow OSHA guidelines.
   d. Turn on the communication systems.

2. Dental stools for dental assistant should be made available that provide for which of the following requirements?

   a. fixed back rest for vertical adjustment
   b. abdominal arm
   c. fixed back rest to support lumbar region
   d. thin seat

3. In what area would the panoramic machine be located?

   a. x-ray processing room
   b. consultation room
   c. treatment room
   d. radiography room

4. How to handle contaminated items falls under rules for

   a. physical safety.
   b. biohazard safety.
   c. chemical safety.

5. What should the assistant always wear when operating rotary equipment?

   a. overgloves
   b. safety eyewear
   c. examination gloves
   d. surgical cap

6. The front delivery systems are located

   a. over the patient's chest and between the dentist and the assistant.
   b. to the right-front of the assistant.
   c. to the right-front of the dentist.
   d. behind the patient's head in front of the assistant.

7. The rheostat is used to

    a. control the air/water syringe.

    b. regulate the water reservoir.

    c. control the speed of the dental handpiece.

    d. control the overhead light.

8. Should the assistant use chair barriers or disinfect the dental chair between patients?

    a. chair barriers

    b. disinfect

    c. dentist's preference

    d. Follow manufacturer's directions.

9. Self-contained water reservoir is filled with _____ water.

    a. tap

    b. drinking

    c. distilled

    d. mouth rinse

10. Which step must be performed first when preparing the treatment for the next patient?

    a. Remove and discard gloves worn during patient treatment.

    b. Don utility gloves.

    c. Cover used tray and transport to sterilization.

    d. Disinfect counter.

11. In what position is the dental chair placed for patient seating?

    a. upright

    b. supine

    c. subsupine

    d. ergonomic

12. What should be run for 30 seconds to clear the lines and bring in fresh water from the reservoir for the next patient?

    a. air/water syringe and handpiece hoses

    b. handpiece hoses and oral evacuator hose

    c. air/water syringe and saliva ejector hose

    d. handpiece hoses and saliva ejector hose

13. When escorting the patient to the treatment room, the assistant should

    a. give the patient directions.

    b. ask the patient to follow.

    c. tell the patient treatment room number.

    d. describe the appearance of the treatment room.

14. The assistant should stand next to the _____ and offer _____ to help the patient to be seated.

    a. back rest; a hand

    b. arm rest; an arm

    c. foot rest; a hand

    d. seat rest; an arm

15. The assistant should place the height of the backrest _____ inches above the dentist's thighs.

    a. 2

    b. 3

    c. 4

    d. 5

16. At what height above the patient's chest should the assistant place the dental light?

    a. 12 inches

    b. 24 inches

    c. 30 inches

    d. 36 inches

17. Why should the assistant and dentist wash hands in front of the patient?

    a. It reduces the chance of cross-contamination.

    b. The sinks are in the treatment room.

    c. It makes patient confident that infection control protocol is followed.

    d. It is a law.

18. When the assistant introduces the dentist to a new patient, which of the following is recommended?

    a. Introduce patient first.

    b. Introduce dentist first.

    c. Introduce elder person first.

    d. There is no preference.

19. Which member of the dental team is most likely to explain procedures to the patient on the day of treatment?

    a. receptionist

    b. business manager

    c. dental assistant

    d. dentist

20. Which member of the dental team makes future appointments and completes the financial arrangements at the dismissal of the patient?

    a. receptionist

    b. assistant

    c. dentist

    d. accountant

21. After the treatment is completed and before the patient is dismissed, all of the following are removed from the unit and placed on the procedure tray EXCEPT the

    a. dental handpiece.

    b. high-volume evacuator tip.

    c. saliva ejector.

    d. air/water syringe tip.

CERTIFICATION REVIEW

1. How is the patient positioned in the dental chair for an oral examination?

    a. subsupine

    b. supine

    c. Trendelenburg position

    d. upright

2. What is the best way to maintain the dental equipment used in the treatment room?

    a. Complete weekly maintenance.

    b. Purchase a service contract.

    c. Develop a detailed service record.

    d. Follow the manufacturer recommendation.

3. The dental assistant is seating the patient. When should they put on their personal protective equipment?

    a. after the patient sits in the chair

    b. before the bib, chair, and dental light are positioned

    c. after the bib, chair, and dental light are positioned

    d. before holding the chart and reviewing the patient treatment

4. When putting on personal protective equipment before patient treatment, which barrier should be put on last?

    a. mask

    b. examination gloves

    c. eyewear

    d. protective clothing

5. What position places the chair back until the patient is almost lying down?

   a. upright
   b. supine
   c. subsupine
   d. Trendelenburg

6. What type of gloves should be worn during operatory cleanup?

   a. sterile
   b. exam
   c. utility
   d. nonlatex

7. Which describes what to do when removing and placing surface covers from dental equipment in the treatment area?

   a. Wear exam gloves at all times.
   b. Wear exam gloves when removing contaminated covers; use clean, bare hands to place new cover.
   c. Wear utility gloves when removing contaminated covers; use exam gloves to place new cover.
   d. Wear utility gloves when removing contaminated covers; wash hands and don exam gloves.

8. The assistant's unit is usually set up with the following instrumentation except for the

   a. air/water syringe.
   b. HVE.
   c. three handpieces.
   d. saliva ejector.

9. Where should the dental assistant place the patient's personal items when seating a patient in the dental treatment room?

   a. the patient's lap
   b. to the left of the chair within reach
   c. on the countertop
   d. in a cabinet within their view

10. Which is the best infection control method for dental instruments that cannot be detached from the dental unit and switches?

    a. Saturate-wipe-saturate with high-level disinfectant.
    b. Saturate-wipe-saturate with intermediate-level disinfectant.
    c. Saturate-wipe-saturate with low-level disinfectant.
    d. Cover with impervious barriers that are changed between each patient.

CHAPTER APPLICATION

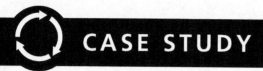

CASE STUDY

The dentist's vision and expectations are reflected in the office design, which should always consider the patients that the dentist serves. The appearance of the dental office makes a statement about the dentist, the dental staff, and the quality of dental care. The reception room, reception desk, and business office are basic components of the office design.

1. What general features should the reception room offer, and how does it affect the patient?

   _____

   _____

   _____

2. Describe the reception desk area and how it is expected to serve the patient.

   _____

   _____

3. Describe the business office and its function.

   _____

   _____

   _____

✖ Critical Thinking

1. While the patient is sitting in the dental chair, the barrier becomes torn. What steps should the dental assistant take?

   _____

   _____

   _____

2. One of the new patients scheduled for the day is a non-English speaking patient. What can the dental team do in advance to make certain they will be able to communicate during the appointment with the patient?

   _____

   _____

   _____

After a long appointment, the patient feels lightheaded as the assistant positions them from the supine to upright position.

1. What is this response called?

_____

_____

2. What should the assistant do to prevent this response?

_____

_____

_____

CHAPTER 19

Dental Instruments and Tray Systems

SPECIFIC INSTRUCTIONAL OBJECTIVES

At the completion of this chapter, you will be able to meet these objectives:

1. Use the terms presented in this chapter.
2. Recall the names, functions, and parts of hand instruments.
3. Describe expendable materials and their uses.
4. Describe types of handpiece power sources.
5. Identify handpiece types, parts, and their use.
6. Compare and contrast the emerging handpieces.
7. Identify the classification of cavities.
8. Name parts of a rotary instrument.
9. Select a rotary instrument appropriate for each type of handpiece.
10. Identify cutting burs by name and number series.
11. Compare and contrast cutting, surgical, vulcanite, and finishing burs.
12. Discuss types of abrasive rotary instruments and mandrels.
13. Compare and contrast care of burs, abrasive rotary instruments, and polishing instruments.
14. Defend need for standardized procedures and tray setups.
15. Describe preparation of tray setups.

VOCABULARY BUILDER

Matching

Match each term with the appropriate definition.

1. _____ chuck
2. _____ carve
3. _____ burnish
4. _____ bur
5. _____ abrasion
6. _____ airotor
7. _____ burlew

a. high-speed handpiece
b. to make smooth
c. abrasive rubber wheel
d. holds rotary instrument
e. shapes restorations by cutting
f. wear down by friction
g. removes decay and shapes tooth structure

8. _____ cauterize
9. _____ carborundum
10. _____ fiber-optic
11. _____ grit
12. _____ serrated
13. _____ tine

a. transmits light to head of handpiece
b. notched surface
c. destroy tissue by burning
d. sharp point
e. abrasive particle size
f. separating disc or Joe Dandy

Fill in the Blank

Please fill in the blank with one of the choices provided.

mandrel	utility	tooth
sequence	cavity preparation	dentist
cavity preparation	handpiece	

1. The dentist completes the _____ using dental instruments to remove caries and diseased tooth structures.

2. The remaining tooth structure after the caries have been removed is called the _____.

3. One end of the _____ holds the rotary instrument, and the other end is inserted into the handpiece.

4. A(an) _____ instrument is made for many uses.

5. The instruments are placed in _____ according to the order the dentist uses them during the procedure.

CHAPTER REVIEW

Matching

Match each hand instrument with its function.

1. _____ hatchet
2. _____ hoe
3. _____ chisel
4. _____ carver
5. _____ burnisher
6. _____ plastic instrument
7. _____ angle former

a. smooths floor of cavity preparation

b. planes the enamel margins of cavity preparation

c. removes weak or undermined enamel

d. smooths condensed amalgam

e. shapes condensed amalgam after preparation has been filled

f. mixes resin material

g. shapes proximal boxes and angle of preparation

Match each part of the bur with its description.

Bur Part

1. _____ shank
2. _____ neck
3. _____ head

Description

a. working end of bur

b. inserted into handpiece

c. tapered connection between other parts

True or False

Circle whether the answer is true or false.

1. **T   F**   The shank is the part of the instrument where the operator grasps or holds the instrument.

2. **T   F**   The high-speed handpiece should be cleaned, lubricated, and sterilized after each patient.

3. **T   F**   A white stone is used when polishing resin restorations.

4. **T   F**   Rubber points have abrasives impregnated into them. They can be sterilized and used several times before they have to be replaced and cannot be sharpened.

5. **T   F**   Sandpaper discs come in x-fine, fine, medium, and coarse grit. They are used to smooth tooth surfaces and resin or plastic restorations.

Multiple Choice

1. _____ instruments are made with aluminum–titanium coating or Teflon.

   a. Liner
   b. Cement

   c. Amalgam
   d. Composite

2. Which of the Black's cavity classifications involves the pits and fissures of teeth?

   a. Class I
   b. Class II
   c. Class III

   d. Class IV
   e. Class V

3. Which of the Black's cavity classification involves the interproximals of anterior teeth?

   a. Class I
   b. Class II
   c. Class III
   d. Class IV
   e. Class V

4. Which statement describes a dental lab bur?

   a. has short shank friction grips
   b. looks like regular cutting burs except larger
   c. looks like regular cutting burs except smaller
   d. used in the patient's mouth

5. Which of the following describes carbide burs?

   a. cuts tooth structures
   b. has different shapes for different types of cuts
   c. numbered for size and shape of the head of the bur
   d. all of these

6. The working end of the instrument may be a

   a. point.
   b. blade.
   c. nib.
   d. all of the above

7. Which instrument is used to remove soft, carious material and has a cutting edge that is rounded all the way around the periphery of the blade?

   a. gingival margin trimmer
   b. carrier
   c. excavator
   d. carver

8. All of these instruments are included in the basic examination setup EXCEPT

   a. excavator.
   b. mouth mirror.
   c. explorer.
   d. cotton pliers.

9. Which instrument's working end is a thin, sharp point of flexible steel?

   a. excavator
   b. cotton pliers
   c. explorer
   d. plastic instrument

10. Which instrument is used to transport and manipulate various materials and is available with either locking or nonlocking handles?

    a. explorers
    b. excavators
    c. cotton pliers
    d. probes

11. What is another name for the low-speed handpiece?

    a. contra angle
    b. right angle
    c. straight handpiece
    d. latch type

12. What will activate and control the speed of the handpiece?

    a. power source
    b. fiber-optic light source
    c. friction
    d. rheostat

13. What was developed to standardize the exact size and angulation of an instrument?

    a. stock number
    b. manufacturer's number
    c. Black's formula
    d. instrument categories

14. Which expendable would be placed in the mouth to control saliva?

   a. cotton gauze square   c. cotton rolls
   b. cotton pellets   d. cotton-tip applicators

15. What part of the bur is held in the handpiece?

   a. head   c. handle
   b. chuck   d. neck

16. Which of the following instruments have abrasive material that may be made of garnet, diamond, and cuttle?

   a. cutting burs   c. discs
   b. fissure burs   d. finishing burs

CERTIFICATION REVIEW

1. An LA37 bur is inserted into which of the following handpieces?

   a. ultrasonic
   b. high-speed
   c. low-speed
   d. laser

2. How do finishing burs differ from cutting burs?

   a. greater variety of shank sizes
   b. greater variety of working lengths
   c. larger circumference
   d. greater number of blades

3. What instrument is used for tactile discovery of decay?

   a. mouth mirror
   b. explorer
   c. periodontal probe
   d. condenser

4. What bur number designates a straight fissure cross cut bur?

   a. 33
   b. 56
   c. 330
   d. 557

5. What category of hand instrument are a hoe, excavator, hatchet, chisel, and gingival margin trimmer?

   a. examination
   b. handcutting
   c. restorative
   d. accessory

6. Which is the required infection control of handpieces between patients?

   a. Saturate-wipe-saturate with intermediate-level disinfectant.
   b. Saturate-wipe-saturate with high-level disinfectant.

c. Clean and submerse in cold disinfectant.

d. Clean and sterilize.

7. All of these are uses for the low-speed handpiece EXCEPT

    a. removes enamel.

    b. defines cavity preparation.

    c. removes soft decay.

    d. smooths composite material.

8. Which handpiece is used to remove calculus and dental cements from the tooth?

    a. low-speed handpiece

    b. laser

    c. ultrasonic

    d. microabrasion

9. All of these are uses for laser handpieces EXCEPT

    a. to cauterize tissue.

    b. for surgical procedures.

    c. bleaching.

    d. removal of amalgam restorations.

10. What rotary instrument is inserted into high-speed handpieces?

    a. short shank latched

    b. short shank friction grip

    c. long shank latched

    d. long shank friction grip

CHAPTER APPLICATION

 ## Critical Thinking

1. The dental assistant should be able to categorize hand instruments when preparing tray setups. Name common handcutting and restorative instruments.

Handcutting instruments: _____

_____

_____

Amalgam restorative instruments: _____

_____

_____

Composite restorative instruments: _____

_____

_____

Image Labeling

1. Identify this instrument:

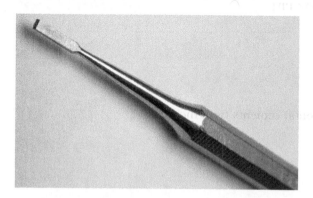

    a. enamel hatchet

    b. straight chisel

    c. gingival marginal trimmer

    d. excavator

2. Identify this instrument:

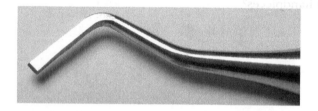

    a. straight chisel

    b. gingival marginal trimmer

    c. enamel hatchet

    d. carver

3. Identify this bur:

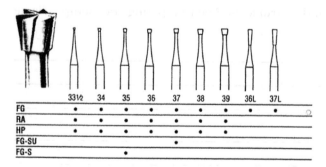

    a. pear

    b. inverted cone

    c. end cutting

    d. round

4. Identify this bur:

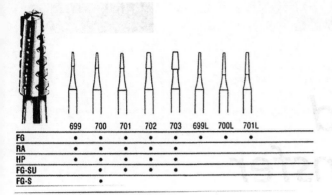

	699	700	701	702	703	699L	700L	701L
FG	•	•	•	•	•	•	•	•
RA	•	•	•	•	•			
HP	•	•	•	•	•			
FG-SU		•	•	•	•			
FG-S		•						

a. wheel

b. inverted cone

c. tapered fissure cross-cut

d. tapered fissure straight

CHAPTER 20

Ergonomics and Instrument Transfer

SPECIFIC INSTRUCTIONAL OBJECTIVES

At the completion of this chapter, you will be able to meet these objectives:

1. Use terms presented in this chapter.
2. Recognize the risk factors that may cause work-related injuries.
3. Describe recommended ergonomics in dentistry.
4. Demonstrate proper positioning for operator, assistant, and patient during four-handed dentistry.
5. Employ motion economy while assisting chairside.
6. Describe team positions, postures, and use of fulcrum in achieving good transfer techniques.
7. Utilize recommended instrument transfer zones.
8. Demonstrate the types of instrument grasps and transfer of instruments for a procedure.
9. Defend the importance of teamwork in four-handed dentistry.

VOCABULARY BUILDER

Matching

Match each term with the appropriate definition.

1. _____ ergo-   a. pressure, burden

2. _____ kinesis   b. work

3. _____ stress   c. place for something

4. _____ –or   d. a thing or person

5. _____ –arium   e. motion

6. _____ carpal   a. draw tight

7. _____ caustic   b. lack of movement

8. _____ flexion   c. capable of burning

9. _____ static   d. bending movement

10. _____ strain   e. wrist

11. _____ armamentarium   a. skilled from experience

12. _____ fulcrum   b. initiate a reaction

13. _____ exchange   c. trade one for another

14. _____ proficient   d. instruments and materials for procedure

15. _____ trigger   e. resting point

CHAPTER REVIEW

True or False

Circle whether the answer is true or false.

1. **T   F**   The use of proper ergonomics saves time and prevents muscle strain and fatigue for the dental team.

2. **T   F**   The way an instrument is grasped also dictates how it is exchanged.

3. **T   F**   The assistant passes and receives instruments with the right hand when working with a right-handed dentist.

4. **T   F**   A smooth transfer of instruments and materials occurs when the assistant is able to anticipate the operator's needs.

5. **T   F**   The dental assistant doesn't transfer dental materials to the dentist.

Matching

Match the term with the best description.

1. _____ transfer zone

    a. a point of rest on which the fingers are stabilized and can pivot

2. _____ fulcrum

    b. the feeling sensed by touch; the pressure of the instrument exchanged in an instrument transfer

3. _____ tactile sensation

    c. the hand that delivers and receives instruments

4. _____ transfer hand

    d. where the assistant brings the instrument to the operator (area just below the patient nose and chin)

Match each grasp type with its definition.

1. _____ pen grasp

    a. provides more control in some procedures

2. _____ palm grasp

    b. grasped in the same manner as a pen or pencil

3. _____ palm-thumb

    c. used with pliers and forceps

4. _____ modified pen

    d. used to hold the evacuation tip in patient's mouth

The one-handed transfer is the most common instrument transfer. Following are the four steps for the instrument transfer. Match each transfer step with its description.

1. _____ signal

    a. Rotate hand toward the operator and place the instrument in the operator's fingers.

2. _____ approach

    b. Lift the instrument from the tray, holding it near the nonworking end.

3. _____ retrieval

    c. Extend the fourth and fifth finger and close around the handle of the instrument.

4. _____ delivery

    d. Operator places hands on either side of patient's face.

Match each transfer zone with its description.

1. _____ Zone A

    a. 12-inch square over patient's chest

2. _____ Zone B

    b. behind and over patient's left shoulder

3. _____ Zone C

    c. below patient's eyes to chin

Match the instrument to the appropriate transfer zone.

1. _____ anesthetic syringe

    a. Zone A

2. _____ hand instrument

    b. Zone B

3. _____ forceps

    c. Zone C

Multiple Choice

1. What may result if the assistant uses repeated, forceful motions of the hand and wrist?

    a. tenosynovitis

    b. lumbosacral neuritis

    c. carpal tunnel syndrome

    d. trapezium strain

2. Proper instrument transfer is accomplished when which of the following is maintained?

   a. The operator's view remains on the oral cavity.

   b. Safety and comfort are maintained for the patient.

   c. Stress and fatigue for the operator and the assistant are reduced.

   d. all of the above

3. Selecting the correct instrument grasp allows

   a. the operator control of the instrument.

   b. greater tactile sensation for the operator.

   c. reduced fatigue for the operator.

   d. all of the above

4. At the beginning of a procedure, the dental assistant places the _____ in the right hand and the _____ in the left hand, and when the dentist puts their hands in position, the dental assistant passes both instruments simultaneously.

   a. cotton pliers; explorer

   b. scissors; explorer

   c. explorer; mouth mirror

   d. mouth mirror; explorer

5. The operator receives the air/water syringe by the

   a. handle.

   b. hose.

   c. tip.

   d. The operator never needs to use the air/water syringe.

6. In what zone are hand instruments transferred?

   a. Zone A

   b. Zone B

   c. Zone C

   d. Zone D

7. How does the operator signal for retrieval of a forceps?

   a. Light the handles of forceps.

   b. Move forceps into Zone B.

   c. Place the forceps on the patient's chest.

   d. Return forceps to the instrument tray.

CERTIFICATION REVIEW

1. Proper ergonomic positioning for the operator's seating includes

   a. feet placed on the foot ring.

   b. elbows close to the body.

   c. thighs angled downward at a 60-degree angle to the floor.

   d. shoulders slightly bent forward.

2. Which describes the proper ergonomic position on the assistant's stool?

   a. thighs angled downward at a 60-degree angle to the floor

   b. feet resting flat on the floor

   c. 4 to 6 inches above the operator

   d. 14 to 16 inches from the patient's oral cavity

3. When the dental assistant is working with a right-handed dentist, what is the 12 to 2 o'clock position called?

   a. operator's zone

   b. static zone

   c. assistant's zone

   d. transfer zone

4. When the dental assistant is working with a right-handed dentist, at what position do they sit to transfer instruments?

    a. 1 to 2 o'clock

    b. 2 to 4 o'clock

    c. 3 to 5 o'clock

    d. 5 to 6 o'clock

5. Which classification of motion involves movement of the fingers and wrist?

    a. I

    b. II

    c. III

    d. IV

6. Once the instrument has been retrieved from the dentist, the instrument should be placed

    a. on top of the patient's bib.

    b. in the holding solution container placed near the tray.

    c. on the tray setup behind any unused instruments.

    d. on the tray setup in its proper order of use.

7. When using the pen grasp single-handed technique, where should the assistant pick up an instrument?

    a. in the middle of the handle

    b. the end closest to the working end

    c. on the end opposite the working end

    d. by the shank of the instrument

8. Which statement describes how to hold the instrument being exchanged for a double instrument exchange using the pen grasp single-handed technique, from the tray to the dentist?

    a. below the instrument in the dentist's hand

    b. over the patient's bib

    c. parallel to the instrument in the dentist's hand

    d. over the patient's left shoulder

9. When transferring instruments with hinges such as forceps and scissors, how should the assistant hold the instrument?

    a. Position the instrument on the bib.

    b. Grasp the handles and pass the instrument to the dentist palm.

    c. Grasp the hinges and direct the handles to the dentist's palm.

    d. Grasp the distal ends of the handles and lay handles on the dentist's palm.

10. How does the dental assistant retrieve an instrument from a right-handed dentist using the single-handed transfer technique?

    a. Use the last finger of the right hand.

    b. Use the last two fingers of the right hand.

    c. Use the last finger of the left hand.

    d. Use the last two fingers of the left hand.

CHAPTER APPLICATION

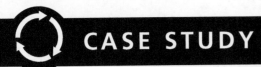

CASE STUDY

A smooth transfer of instruments and materials occurs when the assistant is able to anticipate the operator's needs. Occasionally the assistant will pass the correct instrument but the wrong end.

1. How would the assistant get the desired end into position without placing the instrument back on the instrument tray?

   _____

   _____

   _____

   _____

   _____

   _____

   _____

2. What is the name of this technique?

   _____

   _____

Critical Thinking

1. For the dental assistant, ergonomics is key for comfort and the ability to perform duties effectively and efficiently. List the ways in which the chairside dental assistant can ensure proper positioning.

   _____

   _____

   _____

   _____

   _____

   _____

   _____

2. At the beginning of a procedure, the operator needs the mirror and the explorer to examine the area to be treated. Describe the mirror and explorer transfer for a right-handed operator.

   _____

   _____

   _____

Image Labeling

1. The instrument grasp shown below is called the _____ grasp.

    a. reverse palm-thumb
    b. modified pen
    c. palm-thumb
    d. pen

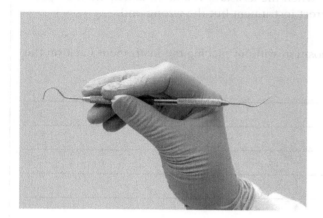

Moisture Control

SPECIFIC INSTRUCTIONAL OBJECTIVES

At the completion of this chapter, you will be able to meet these objectives:

1. Use terms presented in this chapter.

2. Defend the importance of effective moisture control in clinical practice.

3. Select appropriate aspiration technique given a clinical situation.

4. Demonstrate proper positioning and placement of saliva ejector, HVE, and air/water syringe.

5. Select appropriate isolation technique given a clinical situation.

6. Prepare tray setup and the dental dam material for placement.

7. Demonstrate placement of absorbent materials and dental dam.

8. Recall when pharmacological methods are recommended for moisture control.

VOCABULARY BUILDER

Matching

Match each term with the appropriate definition.

1. _____ hemo
2. _____ mal
3. _____ pro
4. _____ prongs
5. _____ gauge
6. _____ septum
7. _____ taut
8. _____ template

a. in favor of
b. thickness of a sheet
c. a pattern
d. blood
e. partition that divides
f. bad
g. tightly drawn
h. pointed part

9. _____ aspirate
10. _____ blanch
11. _____ claustrophobic
12. _____ contour
13. _____ hemostatic
14. _____ impinge
15. _____ invert
16. _____ restoration

a. dental filling
b. curved area
c. stops bleeding
d. to make white
e. remove by suction
f. pinch soft tissue
g. fear of being in closed space
h. turn inward

Fill in the Blank

Please fill in the blank with one of the choices provided.

operative site   lightening strip   aspirate

vasoconstrictor   tenacious   restoration

1. The dentist used a(an) _____ to narrow the blood vessels to slow down the bleeding.

2. The material was very _____ and remained stuck to the surface even after the dentist tried to remove it.

3. The area where treatment is being performed is referred to as the _____.

4. The dentist used a _____ to open the contacts for the placement of the dental dam.

CHAPTER REVIEW

rue or False

Circle whether the answer is true or false.

1. **T F** A dental dam is recommended for infection control because it reduces spatter from dental procedures.

2. **T F** Using one hand for instrument transfer frees the other hand for evacuation.

3. **T F** The reverse palm-thumb grasp (sometimes called the thumb-to-nose grasp) is often used to retract soft tissue while evacuating during a dental procedure.

4. **T F** The only tool needed to maintain moisture control during a dental procedure is the saliva ejector.

5. **T F** OSHA recommends the use of a mask, examination gloves, and protective glasses and protective clothing when using the air/water syringe during a dental procedure.

6. **T F** The HVE has low suction and can be placed under the tongue to control saliva during procedures.

7. **T F** When using the HVE in the maxillary right quadrant, the tip is placed on the facial surface of the teeth.

8. **T F** A cotton pellet is preferred over the air/water syringe to dry deep cavity preparations.

9. **T F** A dental clamp that has an A after its number is used for partially erupted teeth.

10. **T F** A Young's dental dam frame is a complete circle with broad pegs made of radiolucent plastic. It allows for radiographic exposure while placed in the mouth.

Multiple Choice

1. Why is the air/water syringe used during the removal of cotton rolls?

   a. To reduce the tearing the cotton roll
   b. To prevent mucosal tear
   c. To prevent disrupting the restoration
   d. To prolong cotton roll use

2. The ability to maintain the operating field is a critical skill for the dental assistant to obtain. Which of the following skills are essential to oral evacuation tip placement?

   1. The fingers always rest on the occlusal surface.
   2. The evacuator tip is placed approximately one tooth distal to the tooth being worked on.
   3. The bevel of the tip is held parallel to the buccal or lingual surface of the teeth.
   4. The bevel of the tip is parallel to the apex surface of the teeth.
   5. The opening should be even with the occlusal surface.
   6. The primary working end should always be placed toward the cheek.
      a. 1, 5, 6
      b. 2, 3, 5
      c. 2, 3, 6
      d. 1, 3, 5

3. The operator receives the air/water syringe by the

   a. handle.
   b. hose.
   c. tip.
   d. The assistant never transfers the air/water syringe.

4. There are many advantages to using the dental dam, but certain conditions contraindicate its use. Which of the following are contraindications?

   1. provides greater visibility
   2. latex allergies
   3. respiratory congestion
   4. claustrophobic
   5. retracts tongue
   6. provides greater accessibility

       a. 1, 2, 5   c. 2, 3, 4
       b. 2, 3, 6   d. 1, 3, 5

5. Where should the assistant place the HVE when the dentist is using handpiece on the lingual side of the tooth?

       a. on the lingual   c. to the distal
       b. on the facial   d. to the mesial

6. Where should the bevel be placed while evacuating the mouth?

       a. toward the cheek   c. against the gingival tissue
       b. toward the tooth   d. below the occlusal/incisal edge

7. When punching for a Class III preparation on tooth 7, at least how many holes should be punched in the dental dam for placement?

       a. two   c. four
       b. three   d. five

8. When first learning where to place the holes for punching the dental dam, the dental dam can be divided into

       a. thirds.   c. fifths.
       b. fourths.   d. sixths.

9. What should be passed to the operator first to remove the dental dam?

       a. clamp forceps   c. crown and bridge scissors
       b. dental floss   d. Woodson plastic instrument

10. Which is the best technique in placing the dental dam when the cavity to be prepared is a Class V?

       a. clamp before the dental dam   c. dental dam as a unit
       b. clamp after the dental dam   d. the dental dam is not used for a Class V preparation

CERTIFICATION REVIEW

1. When assisting a right-handed dentist, what does the dental assistant do with their right hand when assisting with a procedure?

   a. Transfer instruments.
   b. Retrieve instruments.
   c. Hold the air/water syringe.
   d. Hold the HVE.

2. Which hole number is used to punch for a canine in the placement of a dental dam?

    a. two
    b. three
    c. four
    d. five

3. What food allergies have a connection to latex allergies?

    a. fermentable carbohydrates
    b. milk and cheese
    c. bananas and avocados
    d. grapes and strawberries

4. How should a dry cotton roll be removed from the patient's mouth?

    a. with cotton forceps
    b. Moisten with spray of water.
    c. Retract the lip.
    d. Remove excess moisture with HVE.

5. What device can cause cross-contamination by retraction of infections materials into the patient's mouth if their lips are sealed around it?

    a. a/w syringe
    b. Isolite system
    c. HVE
    d. ejector tip

6. Where should the HVE tip be placed in relation to the tooth being prepared?

    a. anterior
    b. posterior
    c. lingual
    d. mesial

7. Where should the cotton roll be placed when assisting on tooth 3?

    a. lingual to the first molar
    b. next to the first premolar
    c. in the floor of the mouth
    d. facial mucobuccal fold

8. Where should the dental assistant begin spraying the a/w syringe with a full mouth rinse?

    a. maxillary left to right
    b. maxillary right to left
    c. mandibular left to right
    d. mandibular right to left

9. What will prevent saliva from leaking from the punched holes when placing a dental dam?

    a. placing stabilizing cord between the contacts
    b. inverting the edges of the dental dam
    c. punching smaller holes
    d. placing lubricant on the underside of the dental dam

10. How can the assistant prevent the dental clamp from falling into the patient's mouth?

    a. Place stabilizing cord between contacts.

    b. Place a ligature tie around bow of clamp.

    c. Always place dental dam first.

    d. Use a small clamp.

CHAPTER APPLICATION

 CASE STUDY

Rose is scheduled for an amalgam procedure. The patient strongly states that they have never had a dental dam placed in their mouth and that they do not want one. What four advantages can the dental assistant discuss with the patient to explain why the dentist prefers working with a dental dam?

1. _____

_____

_____

2. _____

_____

_____

3. _____

_____

_____

4. _____

_____

_____

Critical Thinking

1. While suctioning the patient's mouth, they stick their tongue against the bevel of the HVE. The tongue becomes stuck in the bevel. What can the assistant do to release the suction from the tongue?

   a. Turn the HVE switch off.

   b. Turn the bevel.

   c. Quickly pull the HVE at a 90-degree angle.

   d. Depress tongue with finger.

2. What three factors should the assistant consider when selecting the clamp for the dental dam procedure?

   a. _____

   b. _____

   c. _____

Image Labeling

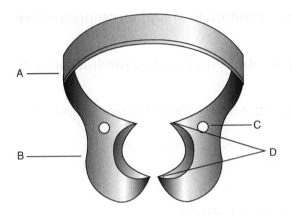

Identify the parts of the dental clamp.

1. A _____

2. B _____

3. C _____

4. D _____

CHAPTER 22

New Patient Examination

SPECIFIC INSTRUCTIONAL OBJECTIVES

At the completion of this chapter, you will be able to meet these objectives:

1. Use terms presented in this chapter.
2. Differentiate between a limited/emergency examination and a comprehensive examination.
3. State the armamentarium necessary for a limited/emergency examination and new patient examination.
4. Discuss the role of the dental assistant during a limited/emergency examination and a new patient examination.
5. Describe forms included in patient's records.
6. Take patient's vitals.
7. Describe dental radiographs taken during examinations.
8. Explain purpose of the extraoral and intraoral soft tissue examination.
9. Describe recording of patient's occlusion and oral habits.
10. Recognize various types of dental charts.
11. Utilize tooth numbering and identification systems.
12. Interpret charting symbols and abbreviations.
13. Discuss the significance of the dental diagnosis.
14. Explain the importance of establishing patient goals when treatment planning.
15. Summarize steps in financial planning.

VOCABULARY BUILDER

Matching

Match each term with the appropriate definition.

1. _____ palpate
2. _____ bruxism
3. _____ attrition
4. _____ baseline
5. _____ periodontal charting
6. _____ atypical
7. _____ examination

a. tooth wear due to tooth contact
b. pocket and sulcus depths are taken
c. inspection
d. examine by touch
e. not normal
f. guideline for comparison
g. habit of grinding teeth

8. _____ appliance
9. _____ denture
10. _____ impacted
11. _____ implant
12. _____ pontic
13. _____ veneer
14. _____ bridge
15. _____ abutment

a. remaining tooth supporting an appliance
b. tooth inserted into the alveolus
c. a device that replaces missing teeth
d. layer of tooth colored material
e. artificial replacement of teeth
f. crowns for teeth on either side of a gap
g. tooth confined in socket
h. artificial tooth attached to an appliance

CHAPTER REVIEW

Matching

Match the tooth condition with the appropriate symbol.

1. _____ dental caries
2. _____ recurrent caries
3. _____ fracture
4. _____ to be extracted
5. _____ abscess

a. outline existing restoration in red
b. circle tooth in red
c. color involved surfaces in red
d. red circle at apex
e. red zig-zag line

Match the treatment with the appropriate symbol.

1. _____ exfoliated primary tooth
2. _____ amalgam restoration
3. _____ composite restoration
4. _____ enamel sealant
5. _____ implant

a. outline involved surface in blue
b. horizontal blue lines through root
c. blue letter "S" on involved surfaces
d. color involved surfaces in solid blue
e. blue X over tooth

Match the cavity classification with the surface area(s).

Classification	Surface Area(s)
1. _____ Class I	a. two or more surfaces posterior
2. _____ Class II	b. interproximal surface of anterior
3. _____ Class III	c. cervical third facial or lingual surface
4. _____ Class IV	d. caries in pits and fissures
5. _____ Class V	e. interproximal surface and incisal edge of anterior

Match the system with its corresponding coding.

System	Corresponding Coding
1. _____ Universal/National	a. 1 for the upper right quadrant
2. _____ Fédération Dentaire Internationale	b. 1–8 in each quadrant
3. _____ Palmer	c. 1–16, 17–32

Match the corresponding charting symbol to the condition/restoration.

1. _____ missing teeth

a.

2. _____ teeth impacted or unerupted

b.
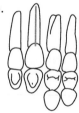

3. _____ teeth that need root-canal therapy

c.
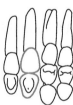

4. _____ tooth with full gold crown

d.

5. _____ tooth with porcelain crown

e.

Multiple Choice

1. Which of the following are required to record on a dental chart the conditions in the patient's oral cavity?

   a. symbols

   b. numbers

   c. colors

   d. all of the above

2. When taking a temperature using a tympanic thermometer, it is placed in/on the patient's

   a. mouth.

   b. forehead.

   c. ear.

   d. armpit.

3. A mother who has never had her daughter (Diedra) seen in the dental office calls complaining that Diedra fell. Diedra has chipped front teeth, and her mouth is bleeding. What should be scheduled for Diedra?

   a. limited oral examination

   b. comprehensive new patient examination

   c. referral to urgent care facility

   d. Deny treatment because she has not been seen in the office previously.

4 The software programs for computer charting(s) can record the following periodontal charting

   a. conditions of dentition.

   b. conditions of occlusion.

   c. conditions of tissue.

   d. all of the above

5. For which purpose(s) would the dentist use an intraoral image?

   a. patient to see their dental problems

   b. for before and after pictures

   c. documentation of treatment

   d. all of the above

6. Why is periodontal probing completed during a new patient examination?

   a. Check for tooth mobility.

   b. Examine suppuration.

   c. Measure pocket depths.

   d. Evaluate root development.

7. What is the purpose of palpating during the intraoral examination?

   a. Evaluate TMJ.

   b. Feel for lumps or bumps.

   c. Locate pathologic lesions.

   d. all of the above

CERTIFICATION REVIEW

1. Angles's classification is used to classify and describe

   a. restorations.

   b. conditions.

   c. types of teeth.

   d. occlusion and malocclusion.

2. When using the universal tooth numbering system, what symbol represents the primary maxillary right central incisor?

   a. D

   b. E

   c. F

   d. G

3. Which represent the numbers used in the universal tooth numbering system for charting the teeth in the mandibular right quadrant?

    a. 1–8

    b. 9–16

    c. 17–24

    d. 25–32

4. What color of symbols indicates that work needs to be done in the patient's clinical records?

    a. black

    b. red

    c. blue

    d. gold

5. What color of symbols is used to chart existing restorations?

    a. black

    b. red

    c. blue

    d. gold

6. When charting using the International Standards Organization system, which symbol represents the mandibular left second molar?

    a. 17

    b. 27

    c. 37

    d. 47

7. During an oral examination, the assistant is responsible for all of the following EXCEPT

    a. assisting patient in completing their medical history.

    b. recording the dentist's finding.

    c. determining future treatment.

    d. preparing patient and room for treatment.

8. Two long blue vertical lines drawn between teeth 8 and 9 on a patient chart would indicate

    a. open contacts.

    b. diastema.

    c. mobility.

    d. has been extracted.

9. What classification of decay is located on the gingival third on the facial or lingual surfaces of teeth?

    a. I

    b. II

    c. III

    d. IV

    e. V

10. A new patient clinical examination consists of all of the following EXCEPT

    a. soft tissue examination.

    b. occlusion classification.

    c. charting of tooth conditions.

    d. dental prophylaxis.

CHAPTER APPLICATION

 CASE STUDY

Since Ester's last dental visit, a change has occurred in her gingival tissue. The following conditions were noted on the chart. Write the name of the teeth where these conditions have been noted.

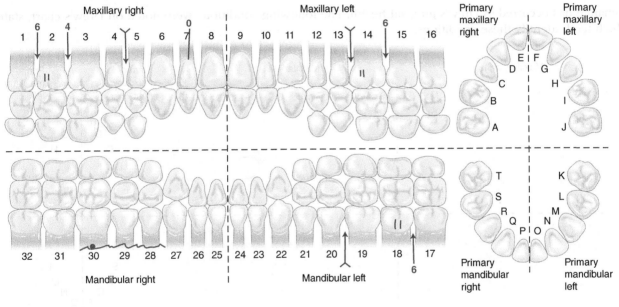

1. root canal

_____

_____

2. abscess

_____

_____

3. periodontal pockets

_____

_____

_____

4. gingival recession

_____

_____

5. gingival furcation involvement

_____

6. mobility

_____

 Critical Thinking

A change has occurred in Drew's gingival health. The following conditions were noted on Drew's chart; state which teeth identify these conditions.

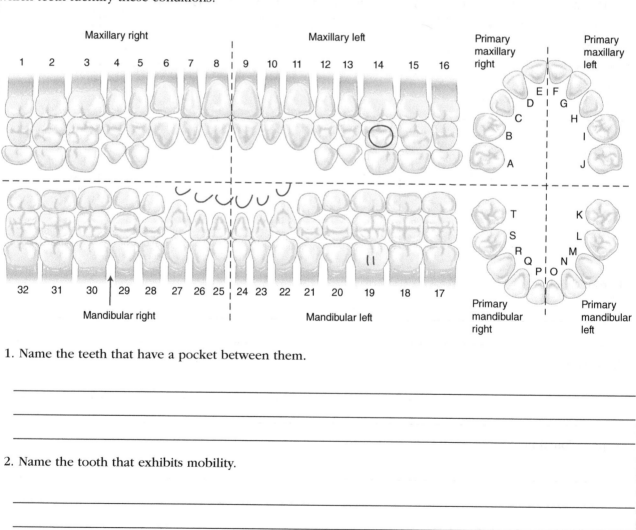

1. Name the teeth that have a pocket between them.

_____

_____

_____

2. Name the tooth that exhibits mobility.

_____

_____

3. Name the tooth and surface that has a temporary restoration.

_____

_____

_____

4. Name the teeth that have heavy calculus.

_____

_____

_____

CHAPTER 23

Anesthesia and Sedation

SPECIFIC INSTRUCTIONAL OBJECTIVES

At the completion of this chapter, you will be able to meet these objectives:

1. Use the terms presented in this chapter.
2. Defend the importance of pain control.
3. Compare and contrast local anesthetics and topical anesthetics.
4. Describe the purpose of non-injectable local anesthetics.
5. State the rationale for vasoconstrictors.
6. Compare and contrast the different concentrations vasoconstrictor in a local anesthetic cartridge.
7. Compare and contrast the three types of dental oral anesthetic techniques.
8. Identify the needle insertion site for the block injections discussed in the chapter.
9. Describe the supplemental local anesthetic techniques.
10. State the rationale for local anesthetic reversal agents.
11. Discuss the advantages of a computer controlled local anesthetic delivery system.
12. Discuss the complications that may occur due to local anesthesia administration.
13. Outline the steps in preventing a medical emergency related to local anesthesia administration.
14. Identify the signs and symptoms of a reaction to epinephrine from a local anesthetic cartridge.
15. List the armamentarium necessary for administration of dental anesthesia.
16. Identify the parts of the local anesthetic syringe.
17. Identify the parts of the local anesthetic cartridge.

18. Identify the parts of the local anesthetic needle.

19. State the correct sequence of steps in assembling a local anesthetic syringe.

20. State what should be included when making a chart entry for local anesthesia administration.

21. Discuss the specifics of the Needlestick Safety Act.

22. Outline the CDC recommendations for postexposure management.

23. Compare and contrast the different types of sedation.

24. State the beneficial effects of nitrous oxide on a patient.

25. List the signs and symptoms of Stage I analgesia.

26. Discuss nitrous oxide–related safety measures.

27. Outline the steps in assisting with nitrous oxide administration.

VOCABULARY BUILDER

Matching

Match each term with the appropriate definition.

1 _____ hematoma

2 _____ pKa

3. _____ topical

4. _____ diffuses

5. _____ permeates

6. _____ diaphragm

7. _____ rubber stopper

8. _____ harpoon

9. _____ gauge

10. _____ titrated

a cover throughout

b. latex rubber membrane

c. harpoon of syringe embeds here

d. diameter of needle lumen

e. sharp end of the plunger

f. clotted blood in tissues

g. administer medication slowly while monitoring effects

h. applied external to the body

i. used to measure acidity of hydrogen

j. spreads

CHAPTER REVIEW

Matching

Match the type of injection with the teeth most affected.

Injection

1. _____ infiltration

2. _____ middle superior alveolar nerve block

3. _____ inferior alveolar nerve block

4. _____ mental nerve block

Effect

a. a mandibular quadrant

b. mandibular premolars, canines, incisors

c. maxillary premolars in one quadrant

d. individual teeth

The type of syringe most commonly used for dental procedures is the aspirating syringe. Recommended by the ADA, it is designed to allow the operator to check the position of the needle before depositing the anesthetic solution. Match the part with its function.

Part

1. _____ thumb ring

2. _____ finger grip

3. _____ harpoon

4. _____ threaded end

Function

a. allows operator to hold syringe

b. barbed tip end that engages the cartridge

c. where the needle attaches to the syringe

d. allows the operator to aspirate

Multiple Choice

1. Which of the following forms are injectable local anesthetics available in?

   a. topical
   b. gas
   c. solution
   d. gel

2. Which of the following is not an amide compound found in local anesthetic solutions?

   a. lidocaine
   b. mepivacaine
   c. prilocaine
   d. procaine

3. Which category of local anesthetic solution provides up to 90 minutes of pulpal anesthesia and up to 3.5 hours of soft tissue anesthesia?

   a. intermediate
   b. long
   c. short
   d. all of the above

4. Which is the vasoconstrictor used in local anesthetic cartridges in the United States?

   a. oxygen
   b. phentolamine mesylate
   c. epinephrine
   d. water

5. Which of the following is not among the most common vasoconstrictor ratios?

   a. 1:200,000
   b. 1:50,000
   c. 1:10,000
   d. 1:100,000

6. Which of the following is defined as the sensation of persistent numbness?

    a. hematoma

    b. paresthesia

    c. trismus

    d. allergy

7. Which of the following injection methods places anesthetic solution in tissue near the small terminal nerve branches?

    a. computerized

    b. local infiltration

    c. field block

    d. nerve block

8. Which of the following injection method deposits local anesthetic near larger terminal nerve branches?

    a. nerve block

    b. computerized

    c. local

    d. field block

9. Which of the following injection methods deposits anesthetic solutions near a main nerve trunk?

    a. field block

    b. computerized

    c. electronic

    d. nerve block

10. Which injection uses a long needle?

    a. infiltration

    b. incisive

    c. mental

    d. infraorbital

11. Which of the following is defined as the slanted tip of the needle?

    a. lumen

    b. gauge

    c. bevel

    d. shank

12. The syringe end of the needle penetrates the anesthetic solution at which location?

    a. aluminum cap

    b. rubber stopper

    c. piston rod

    d. diaphragm

CERTIFICATION

1. Which of the following conditions indicate that the anesthetic cartridge should be discarded?

    a. large bubbles

    b. extruded plunger

    c. corrosion

    d. all of the above

2. What is the best method to recap a needle?

    a. Scoop the needle cover using one hand.

    b. Use a recapping device.

    c. There is no need to recap the needle.

    d. Leave it uncapped on the tray in case it needs to be used again.

3. What color is the nitrous oxide tank?

    a. red

    b. green

    c. blue

    d. yellow

4. Lidocaine with 1:100,000 provides pulpal anesthesia for how long?

   a. 1 to 2 hours

   b. 2 to 3 hours

   c. 30 minutes to 1 hour

   d. 15 minutes

5. Which nerve must be anesthetized to provide anesthesia to the soft tissues of the mandibular molars?

   a. inferior alveolar

   b. mental

   c. incisive

   d. buccal

6. How long should a patient receive 100% oxygen after a procedure involving nitrous oxide sedation has been completed?

   a. Oxygen is not required.

   b. a minimum of 5 minutes

   c. a minimum of 15 minutes

   d. 1 hour

7. Which of the following is a contraindication to nitrous oxide use on a patient?

   a. patient with dental anxiety

   b. patient with a gag reflex

   c. first trimester pregnancy

   d. long appointment

8. Why is it important to use a scavenging system with nitrous oxide sedation?

   a. so the patient receives 100% nitrous oxide

   b. so exposure of the operator to nitrous oxide is minimized

   c. allows patient to be comfortable while receiving treatment

   d. makes time pass quickly

9. Which of the following is not correct regarding local anesthetic overdose?

   a. Reviewing and updating the medical history at each visit is important in preventing a local anesthetic overdose.

   b. Aspirating prior to injecting the local anesthetic is not important in preventing a local anesthetic overdose.

   c. The amount of local anesthetic administered is a factor in determining a local anesthetic overdose.

   d. The rate of injection of local anesthesia is a factor in determining a local anesthetic overdose.

10. Which of the following is not correct regarding nitrous oxide?

   a. Nitrous oxide is a stable, nonflammable gas.

   b. The patient is unable to respond while sedated with nitrous oxide.

   c. Nitrous oxide is administered through a nasal hood.

   d. Nitrous oxide has a sweet smell.

CASE STUDY 1

In charting anesthetic administration for Laura, the following chart notations are made: R-PSANB. Define each symbol.

1. R.

_____

_____

2. PSANB. Define the injection.

_____

_____

3. What is the location for this injection? Which teeth or tissues are affected?

_____

_____

_____

CASE STUDY 2

Most dental procedures require some form of anesthesia. One of the dental assistant's major responsibilities is the care and handling of the equipment to prepare for local anesthetic.

1. What equipment is needed to administer dental local anesthetic?

_____

_____

_____

_____

_____

_____

_____

_____

_____

_____

2. What should the thumb ring be checked for?

_____

_____

3. Describe needle lengths.

_____

_____

_____

_____

4. Explain two cartridge colors and their respective concentrations, with or without epinephrine.

Critical Thinking

1. Needlesticks can occur during transfer of the syringe or during the recap procedure. List the procedure to follow when a needlestick occurs.

_____

_____

_____

_____

_____

_____

_____

_____

_____

_____

_____

_____

_____

_____

2. What are the correct steps in assembling a local anesthetic syringe?

_____

_____

_____

_____

_____

_____

_____

_____

_____

_____

_____

_____

_____

_____

_____

_____

_____

CHAPTER **24**

Dental Prophylaxis and Recare Appointment

SPECIFIC INSTRUCTIONAL OBJECTIVES

At the completion of this chapter, you will be able to meet these objectives:

1. Use terms presented in this lesson.
2. List the six dental hygiene standards of care.
3. Describe the steps of the assessment phase.
4. Identify data collected during periodontal charting.
5. Discuss the role of the dental assistant during comprehensive periodontal charting.
6. Discuss the importance of the dental hygiene diagnosis.
7. List the components of the dental hygiene care plan.
8. Explain the different types of dental hygiene treatment.
9. Identify the functions of the different types of dental hygiene instrumentation.
10. Differentiate between the various types of hand instruments that are used for dental hygiene treatment.
11. Identify a dental hygiene hand instrument by its design for use.
12. Differentiate between the various types of powered instruments that are used for dental hygiene treatment.
13. Recognize contraindications to powered scalers.
14. Determine the method of treatment for sensitivity based on the patient's symptoms.
15. Discuss the role of the dental assistant during dental hygiene instrumentation.
16. Compose postoperative instructions following nonsurgical periodontal therapy.
17. Discuss the importance of the evaluation visit.
18. Document treatment.

VOCABULARY BUILDER

Matching

Match each term with the appropriate definition.

1. _____ scaling

2. _____ root planing

3. _____ prophylaxis

4. _____ debridement

5. _____ sonic

6. _____ piezoelectric

7. _____ magnetostrictive

8. _____ scaler

a. therapeutic instrumentations of the crown and root of the tooth, which includes scaling and root planing

b. smoothing of the root surface of a tooth to promote gingival health

c. removal of biofilm, calculus, and stains from the crown and root surfaces with manual and powered instruments as a preventative measure against oral diseases

d. the removal of calculus, biofilm, and stain on the teeth by means of instruments

e. crystals subject to mechanical stress producing an electric charge

f. a dental instrument used for removal of calculus from teeth

g. Use of vibrations and waves creating a high frequency that is audible to the human ear

h. a material that change shape and dimensions and are used to convert mechanical energy into electromagnetic energy and vice versa

1. _____ sub-

2. _____ supra-

3. _____ peri-

4. _____ phage-

a. around

b. under

c. above

d. eat or devours

CHAPTER REVIEW

True or False

Circle whether the answer is true or false.

1. The assessment portion of the dental hygiene visit is crucial. It covers components of the visit not included in the comprehensive dental exam.

   a. Both statements are true.
   b. Both statements are false.
   c. The first statement is true; the second statement is false.
   d. The first statement is false; the second statement is true.

2. **T   F**   Supragingival scaling is performed above the gumline.

3. Paired instruments are mirrored. This allows the use of one instrument to access the buccal and lingual without having to change instruments.

    a. Both statements are true.

    b. Both statements are false.

    c. The first statement is true; the second statement is false.

    d. The first statement is false; the second statement is true.

4. **T   F**   A preprocedural rinse is only necessary for NSPT.

5. During the oral prophylaxis, setup includes hand scalers. Ultrasonic instrumentation is used for NSPT and not the oral prophylaxis.

    a. Both statements are true.

    b. Both statements are false.

    c. The first statement is true; the second statement is false.

    d. The first statement is false; the second statement is true.

Multiple Choice

1. Place the following components of dental hygiene care in order:

    1. planning

    2. assessment

    3. evaluation

    4. dental hygiene diagnosis

    5 documentation

    6. implementation

    a. 1, 3, 6, 2, 5, 4   c. 4, 1, 3, 2, 6, 5

    b. 2, 1, 3, 4, 6, 5   d. 2, 1, 6, 4, 3, 5

2. Which of the following does not belong on the oral prophylaxis tray?

    a. ultrasonic tip   c. Columbia 13/14

    b. Gracey 13/14   d. sickle scalers

3. The ADHA updated its standards of clinical dental hygiene practice to include the dental hygiene diagnosis (DHDx) in which year?

    a. 1975   c. 2001

    b. 1990   c. 2016

4. Which of the following is NOT true of area-specific curets?

    a. designed to go subgingivally   c. two instruments required to scale an entire quadrant

    b. have two working cutting edges   d. have a longer shank

5. Dentinal hypersensitivity is due to which of the following?

    a. excess enamel   c. gingival overgrowth

    b. exposure of dentin   d. excess dentin

6. Which of the following is NOT a risk factor for caries?

    a. excess saliva   c. inadequate sources of topical fluoride

    b. poor oral hygiene   d. diet and high fermentable carbohydrates

7. Which of the following is a risk factor for periodontal disease?

    a. diabetes

    b. anemia

    c. diet high in fiber

    d. seasonal allergies

8. Which of the following is considered a healthy sulcus?

    a. 0–3 mm

    b. 0–4 mm

    c. 0–5 mm

    d. 0–6 mm

9. How many measurements are on each tooth?

    a. 3

    b. 4

    c. 6

    d. 8

10. One contraindication to ultrasonic scaling is _____.

    a. too much calculus

    b. not enough calculus

    c. diabetes

    d. respiratory diseases

11. The component of the dental hygiene visit that includes the health history, radiographs, and dental charting is the _____.

    a. assessment

    b. dental hygiene diagnosis

    c. evaluation

    d. implementation

12. During the comprehensive periodontal charting, the first step the operator completes is to _____.

    a. examine for suppuration

    b. measure periodontal depth

    c. examine for missing teeth

    d. examine for bleeding

13. During scaling and root planing, the conservation of _____ is necessary.

    a. enamel

    b. dentin

    c. pulp

    d. cementum

14. The sickle scaler has a _____ cross-section.

    a. triangular

    b. circular

    c. semicircular

    d. hexagonal

15. When measuring for clinical attachment level, you need to _____ if the tissue is grown over the CEJ.

    a. add

    b. subtract

    c. divide

    d. multiply

16. A Nabers probe is designed to measure which of the following?

    a. bleeding

    b. furcation

    c. clinical attachment level

    d. mobility

Matching

Match each term with the appropriate definition.

1. _____ anterior sickle

2. _____ Columbia 13/14

3. _____ Gracey 1/2

4. _____ Gracey 13/14

    a. simple shank, used on crowns only

    b. simple shank, rounded back allowing subgingival use

    c. complex shank rounded back allowing subgingival use

    d. complex shank, used anterior and posterior, truly universal

CERTIFICATION REVIEW

Multiple Choice

1. Which of the following instruments would be found on the tray setup for root planing?

   a. elevator

   b. scalpel

   c. universal curet

   d. burnisher

2. Which of the following instruments is used for tactile discovery of calculus?

   a 11/12 explorer

   b. 23 explorer

   c. Nabers probe

   d. scaler

3. What symbols are used to identify furcation on paper charting?

   a. circles

   b. triangles

   c. squares

   d. lines

4. When setting up a tray for comprehensive periodontal charting, which of the following is NOT included?

   a. Nabers probe

   b. mouth mirror

   c. cotton forceps

   d. HVE

5. Which powered instrument moves in a linear pattern?

   a. sonic

   b. ultrasonic

   c. piezoelectric

   d. magnetostrictive

6. For a patient with dentinal hypersensitivity, which of the following at-home treatments could be recommended?

   a. 5% potassium nitrate

   b. cool saltwater rinses

   c. whitening toothpaste

   d. triclosan

7. Topical desensitizing agents can be delivered in the form of all of the following EXCEPT

   a. liquid

   b. paste

   c. varnish

   d. tablet

8. Chlorhexidine rinses may be indicated for which procedure?

   a. scaling and root planing

   b. periodontal charting

   c. oral prophylaxis

   d. new patient exam

9. Which instrument is not designed to be used on recession?

   a. Gracey 1/2

   b. Columbia 13/14

   c. ODU 11/12 explorer

   d. sickle scaler

10. Thinner ultrasonic tips are designed for what type of use?

    a. supragingival scaling

    b. intrinsic stain removal

    c. light calculus removal

    d. moderate to heavy calculus

CHAPTER APPLICATION

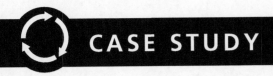

CASE STUDY

Evelin is scheduled for a scaling and root planing visit. She is a 50-year-old female in good health. She has a history of periodontal disease, and the comprehensive perio chart shows pocket depths up to 7 mm. It has been decided to use adjunctive therapy in any pockets 5 mm and deeper.

1. What is adjunctive therapy?

_____

_____

_____

2. How is it decided how many quadrants will be treated in the same day?

_____

_____

_____

3. In which component of dental hygiene care would the operator decide if the initial treatment was successful?

_____

_____

4. If treatment was not successful, what would be the next step?

_____

_____

Image Labeling

Questions 1–3: Label the following instruments by design.

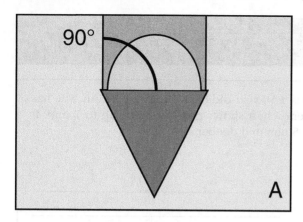

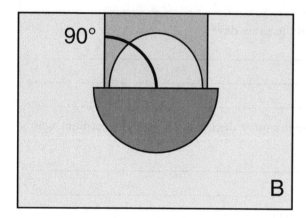

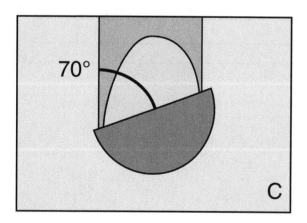

1. _____ sickle scaler

2. _____ area-specific curet

3. _____ universal curet

CHAPTER 25

Coronal Polishing and Fluoride Application

SPECIFIC INSTRUCTIONAL OBJECTIVES

At the completion of this chapter, you will be able to meet these objectives:

1. Use terms presented in this lesson.
2. State the rationale for coronal polishing.
3. Explain the contraindications for coronal polish.
4. Differentiate between intrinsic and extrinsic stain and state the cause of each.
5. Indicate the appropriate type of polishing method.
6. State the rationale for selective polishing.
7. Describe the rationale for each step in the coronal polish procedure.
8. Identify proper ergonomics while coronal polishing.
9. Choose the correct attachment for coronal polishing.
10. Determine the type of abrasive necessary based on individual need.
11. Describe the technique for air-powder polishing.
12. Explain the types of equipment and materials used to perform a coronal polish.
13. Describe the indications for professional topical fluoride.
14. State the types of topical fluoride available for a professional applied fluoride treatment.
15. Summarize the steps in the fluoride tray application.
16. Describe the characteristics of an ideal fluoride tray.
17. Summarize the steps in the fluoride varnish application.
18. Justify use of fluoride varnish over fluoride tray application.
19. Discuss indications for use of silver diamine fluoride.
20. Recognize the formulation of silver diamine fluoride and distinguish the purpose of each ingredient.
21. List steps in application of silver diamine fluoride.

VOCABULARY BUILDER

Matching

Match each term with the appropriate definition.

1. _____ exogenous
2. _____ endogenous
3. _____ abrasive
4. _____ intrinsic
5. _____ humectant
6. _____ substantivity
7. _____ prophy brush
8. _____ polishing
9. _____ off-label use
10. _____ fulcrum
11. _____ extrinsic
12. _____ chromogenic
13. _____ topical fluoride application

a. a substance used for abrading, smoothing, or polishing
b. producing color or pigment
c. produced within or caused by factors within the organism
d. originating or produced outside of the organism
e. originating or acting from outside
f. point of stabilization for instrumentation with the ring finger
g. an agent that promotes retention of moisture
h. originating or acting from inside
i. a drug used to treat a condition for which it has not been officially approved
j. to make smooth and glossy, usually by friction
k. made with nylon bristles to fit into the dental grooves and pits
l. property of continuing therapeutic action despite removal of vehicle
m. a fluoride applied directly to the teeth

CHAPTER REVIEW

Multiple Choice

1. The rubber cup used in polishing should have all of the following qualities EXCEPT being

   a. soft.
   b. rough.
   c. flexible.
   d. adaptable to contours.

2. These are used with polishing agents to polish deep occlusal grooves and pits.

   a. prophy brushes
   b. soft wooden points
   c. abrasive strips
   d. bridge threaders

3. Which of the following describes the polishing stroke when using the rubber cup?

   a. short, continuous, overlapping stroke
   b. long, flowing, continuous stroke
   c. short, intermittent, overlapping stroke
   d. long, intermittent, continuous stroke

4. All of the following are true statements about prophy brushes EXCEPT that they

   a. come in several styles.
   b. are available only with a flat end.
   c. are available in nylon or natural bristles.
   d. come with a snap-on or screw-on end to attach to the prophy angle.

5. When performing the coronal polishing procedure, which is true when using the prophy brush?

    a. Establish a fulcrum four to five teeth away.

    b. No prophy paste is needed.

    c. Soak the brush in cool water.

    d. Place brush bristles in central fossa and move toward the cusp.

6. When air-powder polishing, the sodium bicarbonate polishing agent is contraindicated in patients with which condition?

    a. diabetes

    b. high blood pressure

    c. arthritis

    d. epilepsy

7. Which type of air-powder polishing agent is approved for subgingival use?

    a. glycine

    b. sodium bicarbonate

    c. aluminum trihydroxide

    d. pumice

8. All of the following will affect the rate of abrasion EXCEPT

    a. speed.

    b. pressure.

    c. amount of abrasive.

    d. rubber cup size.

Matching

1. _____ stannous fluoride

2. _____ acidulated phosphate fluoride

3. _____ neutral sodium fluoride

4. _____ silver diamine fluoride

a. short shelf life, bitter tasting, can cause staining

b. safe for use in restorations

c. contraindicated for use on restorations

d. can be used to arrest decay in certain circumstances

True or False

Circle whether the answer is true or false.

1. **T F** The coronal polish procedure involves removing soft deposits and extrinsic stains from the surfaces of the teeth and restorations.

2. **T F** The coronal polish is polishing the clinical crown of the tooth. The clinical crown may vary in length.

3. **T F** The coronal polish procedure is contraindicated on patients with hypersensitive teeth.

4. **T F** For caries arrest, silver diamine fluoride should be applied one to two times per year.

5. **T F** Unlike topical fluoride gels or foams, there is little systemic uptake of fluoride varnish, so the chance of systemic toxicity is negligible.

6. When performing coronal polishing, place the rubber cup at a 45-degree angle. Activate the handpiece before the cup touches the tooth.

    a. Both statements are true.

    b. Both statements are false.

    c. The first statement is true; the second statement is false.

    d. The first statement is false; the second statement is true.

7. When using the air-powder polisher, the handpiece tip is held 1–2 mm away from the tooth surface. The tip should placed on the surface for 5 seconds before moving to the next area.

   a. Both statements are true.

   b. Both statements are false.

   c. The first statement is true; the second statement is false.

   d. The first statement is false; the second statement is true.

8. Flour of pumice is used to remove stains from enamel. It is not used on exposed dentin, tooth-colored restorations, or gold restorations because of its high abrasiveness.

   a. Both statements are true.

   b. Both statements are false.

   c. The first statement is true; the second statement is false.

   d. The first statement is false; the second statement is true.

CERTIFICATION REVIEW

Multiple Choice

1. What should be done to increase the uptake of fluoride prior to applying topical fluoride with the tray application?

   a. Moisten the teeth with water.

   b. Have the patient rinse with mouthwash.

   c. Remove biofilm.

   d. Remove calculus.

2. Which of the following is a contraindication of coronal polishing?

   a. diabetes

   b. heart disease

   c. communicable disease

   d. brown stain

3. Tetracycline stain is considered which type of stain?

   a. endogenous

   b. extrinsic

   c. exogenous

   d. chromogenic

4. Which of the following is true when using a fulcrum during a coronal polish?

   a. Use the index finger to fulcrum.

   b. Tooth structure provides the most stable fulcrum.

   c. Soft tissue is not used as a fulcrum.

   d. The pinky will rest lightly on the handpiece.

5. When air-powder polishing on the anterior teeth, angle the nozzle to which degree?

   a. 0 degrees
   b. 30 to 60 degrees
   c. 80 degrees
   d. 90 degrees

6. After eruption, exposure of the tooth to topical fluoride will result in high levels of fluoride at which surface?

   a. deeper
   b. inner
   c. outer
   d. the entire tooth

7. There are fewer clinical trials demonstrating the effectiveness of which type of fluoride delivery?

   a. gel
   b. foam
   c. varnish
   d. rinse

8. Which fluoride is contraindicated in patients with restorations?

   a. neutral sodium fluoride
   b. acidulated phosphate fluoride
   c. stannous fluoride
   d. fluoride varnish

9. It is recommended that a tray fluoride application be applied to the teeth for how many minutes?

   a. 1
   b. 2
   c. 3
   d. 4

10. When applying the fluoride varnish, the patient should be in which position?

    a. supine
    b. semisupine
    c. sitting upright
    d. Trendelenburg

CHAPTER APPLICATION

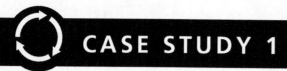

CASE STUDY 1

The dental assistant is preparing to perform a coronal polish on Simon, who has no restorations and is not receiving sealants today. Simon complains of some generalized sensitivity and has minimal to no stains.

1. What should the assistant take into account when selecting a polishing agent for Simon?

   _____

   _____

2. What would be the best selection for the paste to be used on Simon?

   _____

   _____

CASE STUDY 2

During the coronal polishing appointment, the dental assistant notices the patient has a severe gag reflex. The patient has a history of restorations. When it comes time to place the fluoride, the dental assistant chooses to apply a fluoride varnish rather than using the tray technique to avoid any additional gagging.

1. What is the percentage and type of fluoride available in a varnish?

   _____

   _____

2. Why did the assistant choose to apply a fluoride varnish rather than using acidulated phosphate fluoride for the one minute option?

   _____

   _____

3. What are the advantages of fluoride varnish when compared to the tray application?

   _____

   _____

   _____

4. What are the postoperative instructions for the fluoride varnish?

   _____

   _____

   _____

Critical Thinking

1. For the coronal polish procedure, a low-speed dental handpiece is used. List key points and methods for using the dental handpiece that help to avoid operator fatigue.

_____

_____

_____

_____

2. Stains are discoloration of the teeth and are caused by many things. The dental assistant will evaluate stains and determine whether the stains can be removed. Explain intrinsic versus extrinsic stains and exogenous versus endogenous stains.

_____

_____

_____

Image Labeling

Identify the following attachments and accessories in the figure.

1. Assortment of cups, brushes, and points _____

2. Contra-angle with latch _____

3. Disposable prophy angle cup _____

4. Latch brush _____

5. Screw-on prophy cup _____

6. Prophy angle head screw-on _____

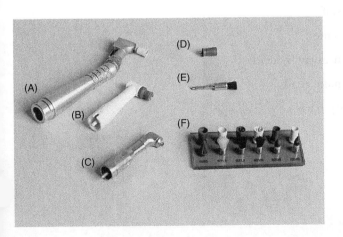

CHAPTER 26

Dental Sealants

SPECIFIC INSTRUCTIONAL OBJECTIVES

At the completion of this chapter, you will be able to meet these objectives:

1. Use terms presented in this chapter.
2. Explain how dental sealants are an important part of a preventive program.
3. List indications and contraindications for dental sealants.
4. Compare and contrast the types of sealant materials.
5. Discuss safety concerns during placement of dental sealants.
6. Recall steps in placing a dental sealant.
7. Determine the cause of sealant failure.

VOCABULARY BUILDER

Matching

Match each term with the appropriate definition.

1. _____ auto
2. _____ poly
3. _____ -ize
4. _____ etch
5. _____ photo
6. _____ prime
7. _____ slurry

a. light
b. thin mixture of substances
c. by self
d. to make
e. wear away by acid
f. to make ready
g. many parts

8. _____ bond	a. thick adhesive
9. _____ cure	b. made of separate parts
10. _____ composite	c. chemical used to make small openings
11. _____ etchant	d. hold together
12. _____ opaque	e. set or harden a material
13. _____ photopolymerize	f. to combine parts by light
14. _____ viscous	g. prevents passage of light

Fill in the Blank

Please fill in the blank with one of the choices provided.

radiometer   sealant

all of these   retention

1. A(an) _____ is applied to surfaces of molars to prevent tooth decay.

2. A(an) _____ resin polymerizes with heat.

3. The tooth is etched for added _____ to hold the sealant in place.

4. A _____ is used to make certain the curing light is functioning properly.

▶CHAPTER REVIEW

True or False

Circle whether the answer is true or false.

1. **T F** After the tooth is etched, rinsed, and dry, it should appear dull and chalky white.

2. **T F** Place the sealant on the distal side of the tooth and allow it to flow to the mesial side of the tooth.

3. **T F** Use a firm scrubbing motion when applying the dental sealant to the enamel surface.

4. **T F** Once the sealant is placed and light-cured, use an explorer to check the hardness and whether the surface is smooth.

5. **T F** Use flour of pumice or nonfluoride prophy paste with a rubber cup or bristle brush to clean the occlusal surface just before placing the sealant material.

Matching

Match each term with the appropriate definition.

1. _____ phosphoric acid	a. self-curing or autopolymerization
2. _____ chemically cured	b. used to open up deep occlusal pits
3. _____ slurry of pumice	c. used as an etchant
4. _____ fissureotomy bur	d. used for isolation of the teeth
5. _____ Garmers clamps	e. used to clean surface of teeth

Multiple Choice

1. Which of the following apply to sealants?

   a. prevent tooth decay

   b. cost less than a restoration

   c. less painful than a restoration

   d. all of the above

2. Which of the following is recognized as an effective means to prevent cavities and to prevent the initiation and progression of early carious lesions of occlusal surfaces of teeth?

   a. application of fluorides

   b. dental sealants

   c. toothbrushing and flossing

   d. mouth rinses

3. _____ sealant material is known as self-cure or autopolymerization.

   a. Light-cured

   b. Mechanical

   c. Heat-cured

   d. Chemically cured

4. The enamel surface is "etched" in preparation for sealant. Application time varies from _____ seconds.

   a. 30 to 60

   b. 30 to 90

   c. 5 to 30

   d. 15 to 30

5. After sealants are placed, the patient is instructed to have them checked once every

   a. 2 years.

   b. 6 months to a year.

   c. 5 years.

   d. Sealants don't need to be checked.

6. The height for holding the curing light is _____ mm directly above the occlusal surface.

   a. 1

   b. 2

   c. 3

   d. 4

7. The sealant procedure area is kept dry by:

   a. asking the patient to keep the tongue still.

   b. placing cotton rolls on both the buccal and of the maxillary lingual surfaces of the mandibular.

   c. placing cotton rolls on the buccal surface.

   d. all of the above

8. The dentist determines the placement of dental sealants by:

   a. their professional judgment.

   b. ADA and CDC guidelines.

   c. the patient's needs and preference on where and when sealants are placed.

   d. all of the above

9. All of the following are used to examine the pit and fissure surfaces *except*

   a. an explorer.

   b. x-rays.

   c. a spoon excavator.

   d. a mouth mirror.

10. This type of sealant material does not need an etchant and continues to release fluoride for up to 2 years.

    a. dental composite resin

    b. glass ionomer

    c. both of the above

    d. neither of the above

11. All of the following are true statements about dental composite resins (BIS-GMA) *except*

    a. they are the most commonly used.

    b. these composites are unfilled or filled.

    c. the unfilled resins are more viscous.

    d. the dental composite resins require no mixing.

12. All of the following are true statements about the color-changing sealants *except*

    a. they assist in evaluating the placement of the resin.

    b. they are tinted red or blue on initial application.

    c. after the initial application they change to opaque white.

    d. they indicate when the sealant is adequately cured.

13. The glass ionomer sealant materials:

    a. bond mechanically to the tooth.

    b. need to be placed in a completely dry environment.

    c. bond directly to the tooth surface.

    d. are more fluid than the composite resins.

14. What is the procedure if the sealant becomes contaminated with saliva during placement?

    a. Nothing needs to be done; the procedure is completed.

    b. The etching procedure must be redone before sealant.

    c. Another layer of sealant is placed, but the tooth does not need to be re-etched.

    d. Using the air/water syringe, wash the area and then place the sealant.

15. The order of steps in placing a dental sealant is:

    a. isolation, etching, pumicing, occlusal evaluation, placement of sealant, polymerization.

    b. pumicing, isolation, etching, placement of sealant, polymerization, occlusal evaluation.

    c. occlusal evaluation, pumicing, isolation, etching, placement of sealant, polymerization.

    d. none of the above

CERTIFICATION REVIEW

1. What is the primary advantage of placing a dental sealant?

    a. prevent interproximal caries

    b. prevent occlusal pits and fissures caries

    c. prevent facial and lingual caries

    d. all of the above

2. What is the primary cause of failure of pit and fissure etched surfaces?

    a. application of the sealant

    b. excessive polishing

    c. curing for too long

    d. moisture contamination

3. The correct sequence of steps for placing a dental sealant is:

    a. isolate area, etch surface, clean with pumice, cure resin, place resin.
    b. clean with pumice, isolate area, etch surface, place resin, cure resin.
    c. isolate area, etch surface, clean with pumice, place resin, cure resin.
    d. clean with pumice, isolate area, place resin, cure resin, etch surface.

4. All of the following would be included in the tray setup for a sealant application *except*

    a. flour of pumice.
    b. microbrush.
    c. primer.
    d. abrasive strips.

5. After which step is it important to keep the tooth surface free of moisture?

    a. pumicing the tooth
    b. placing the cotton rolls
    c. etching the tooth
    d. curing the sealant

6. What is the appearance of a properly etched tooth surface?

    a. frosty
    b. wet
    c. rough
    d. dry

7. The purpose of etching dentin is to remove the:

    a. smear layer.
    b. cementum.
    c. enamel.
    d. biofilm.

8. Who needs to wear light-curing protective eyeglasses when the dental sealant is photopolymerized?

    a. operator
    b. dental assistant
    c. patient
    d. all of the above

9. When is a dental sealant contraindicated on a tooth?

    a. The tooth has been present for years without caries.
    b Decay is present in the tooth.
    c. The patient is allergic to methacrylate.
    d. all of the above

10. Which is most commonly used as the dental sealant material?

    a. dental cement
    b. resin based cement
    c. glass ionomer
    d. amalgam

CHAPTER APPLICATION

 ## Critical Thinking

1. In some states, dental assistants may perform the duty of placing sealants. The most likely cause of sealant failure is lack of moisture control. Describe ways that moisture control can be achieved during sealant placement.

_____

_____

2. Dental sealants have proven to be an effective way to reduce dental decay. List when dental sealants are indicated.

_____

_____

_____

_____

CASE STUDY 1

Serena has several newly erupted permanent mandibular molars. At her routine dental exam, the dentist recommends sealants be placed on the occlusal surfaces of those teeth.

1. How old do you think Serena is?

_____

_____

2. Discuss the best time to place dental sealants.

_____

_____

3. Describe the appearance of teeth that are good candidates for dental sealants.

_____

_____

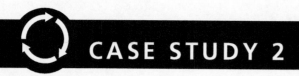

CASE STUDY 2

When placing composite resin sealants, the tooth must be etched so the material will adhere or bond to the enamel surface. Phosphoric acid is routinely used as an etchant for this purpose. Many sealants are set using a curing light.

1. List the safety precautions when using the etchant for sealant placement.

_____

_____

_____

_____

2. List the safety precautions when using the curing light.

_____

_____

_____

SECTION 6

Dental Radiography

Introduction to Dental Radiography, Radiographic Equipment, and Radiation Safety

SPECIFIC INSTRUCTIONAL OBJECTIVES

At the completion of this chapter, you will be able to meet these objectives:

1. Use the terms presented in this chapter.
2. Discuss the purpose of dental radiographs.
3. Identify the person who discovered the x-ray.
4. Define radiation.
5. List the characteristics of electromagnetic radiation.
6. Compare and contrast x-rays with long wavelengths and short wavelengths.
7. Discuss ionization.
8. Compare and contrast the indirect theory of injury and the direct theory of injury.
9. Compare and contrast the different types of interaction that can take place with x-rays.
10. Discuss the components of the dental x-ray machine.
11. State the steps in the production of dental radiographs.
12. Compare and contrast the impact of each of the machine settings on x-ray production.
13. Differentiate among the four types of radiation produced.
14. Define the qualities of a diagnostic image.
15. Discuss the five principles of shadow casting.
16. Describe the principles of ALARA.

17. Differentiate among the units of radiation measurement.
18. Differentiate between the somatic effects and genetic effects of radiation.
19. Compare and contrast between radiosensitive and radioresistant cells.
20. Compare and contrast the occupational exposure and nonoccupational exposure maximum permissible dose.
21. Discuss the nonlinear, nonthreshold curve.
22. State the purpose of intraoral dental films.
23. Discuss the composition of intraoral dental film.
24. Differentiate between radiolucent and radiopaque areas.
25. Define film speed.
26. State the purpose of each intraoral image receptor size.
27. Describe the components of the intraoral film packet.
28. Identify the purposes of extraoral images.
29. Identify the purposes of duplicating film.

VOCABULARY BUILDER

Matching

Match each term with the appropriate definition.

1. _____ dental film		a. acetate sheet that must be chemically processed to produce an image
2. _____ digital sensor		b. energy that is emitted by accelerating particles
3. _____ latent		c. negative end of x-ray tube
4. _____ penumbra		d. positive end of x-ray tube
5. _____ photon		e. negatively charged particles
6. _____ cathode		f. distance between peaks of adjacent waves
7. _____ anode		g. used to capture image, which is viewed on computer
8. _____ electromagnetic radiation		h. shadowy margin around an object
9. _____ wavelength		i. make up all matter
10. _____ atoms		j. an image that will be revealed later
11. _____ electron		k. directs electrons to anode
12. _____ neutron		l. spot on tungsten targets where electrons strike
13. _____ proton		m. radiation absorbed by a substance
14. _____ focusing cup		n. positively charged particles
15. _____ focal spot		o. particles with no charge

16. _____ collimator   p. restructures beam
17. _____ rad   q. rapidly dividing cells
18. _____ radiosensitive cells   r. monitors radiation exposure
19. _____ radioresistant cells   s. particle representing electromagnetic radiation
20. _____ dosimeter   t. cells that rarely divide

CHAPTER REVIEW

Matching

Match each type of radiation with the best definition.

Type

1. _____ primary
2. _____ secondary
3. _____ scatter
4. _____ leakage

Definition

a. escapes in all directions
b. formed when primary x-ray strikes the patient or contacts matter
c. central beam that comes from the x-ray tubehead
d. deflected from its path as it strikes matter

Match each x-ray tube component with its respective function.

Component

1. _____ cathode
2. _____ molybdenum cup
3. _____ filter
4. _____ central beam
5. _____ collimator

Function

a. directs the flow of x-rays
b. solid metal; made of aluminum
c. lead plate
d. negative side where electrons will originate
e. x-rays with short wavelengths

Multiple Choice

1. Who was the professor of physics who discovered x-rays?

   a. Kells   c. Walkoff
   b. Roentgen   d. Rollins

2. What is the name of the open-ended tube that is connected to the tubehead and directs the x-ray beam toward the object to be radiographed?

   a. position indicator device (PID)   c. radiation absorbed dose (rad)
   b. maximum permissible dose (MPD)   d. Roentgen equivalent man (rem)

3. In addition to x-rays, other forms of electromagnetic energy include which of the following?

   a. radio waves   c. visible light
   b. television waves   d. all of the above

4. What is the process by which atoms change into negatively or positively charged ions during radiation?

   a. impulse

   b. milliamperage

   c. kilovoltage

   d. ionization

5. Which of the following is *NOT* a characteristic of high energy wavelengths?

   a. high frequency

   b. low penetrating power

   c. high penetrating power

   d. short wavelength

6. A _____ equals the amount of radiation that will ionize one cubic centimeter of air.

   a. rad

   b. Roentgen

   c. rem

   d. GY

7. The _____ is an abbreviation for the radiation dose to which body tissues are exposed, which is measured in terms of its estimated biological effects.

   a. Sievert

   b. Roentgen

   c. Gray

   d. milliroentgen

8. What is the period between radiation exposure and the development of biological effects called?

   a. radiosensitivity

   b. Sievert

   c. latency

   d. Roentgen

9. Where are the controls of the dental x-ray unit located?

   a. extension arm

   b. x-ray tube

   c. machine head

   d. control panel

10. What is the most common setting for the kilovoltage?

    a. 30

    b. 70 to 90

    c. 10 to 15

    d. 30 to 59

11. What is the most common setting for the milliamperage?

    a. 10 to 15

    b. 30 to 50

    c. 70 to 90

    d. 20 to 40

CERTIFICATION REVIEW

Multiple Choice

1. What is the type of radiation that exits from the x-ray tubehead?

   a. leakage

   b. primary

   c. scatter

   d. secondary

2. What type of radiation forms when the primary x-ray strikes or contacts any type of matter (solid, liquid, or gas)?

   a. leakage

   b. primary

   c. scatter

   d. secondary

3. Electromagnetic radiation with short wavelengths and high frequency have what type of energy?

   a. less
   b. more
   c. magnetic
   d. kinetic

4. Which of the following is the degree of darkness on a radiographic image?

   a. density
   b. contrast
   c. obscureness
   d. opacity

5. What characteristic of a wavelength categorizes its electromagnetic energy?

   a. frequency
   b. peak
   c. length
   d. ionization

6. Which of the following is the least radiosensitive?

   a. bone marrow
   b. thyroid
   c. muscle
   d. lymphoid

7. Which of the following protects the film from scatter radiation?

   a. outer wrapping
   b. black paper
   c. lead foil
   d. none of the above

8. Which of the following film image receptor sizes is the smallest?

   a. 0
   b. 1
   c. 2
   d. 3

9. Which of the following image receptor sizes is used for occlusal exposures on an adult?

   a. 1
   b. 2
   c. 3
   d. 4

10. Which of the following is correct if the operator is using an 8 inch PID as opposed to a 16 inch PID?

    a. The exposure time needs to be increased.
    b. The exposure time needs to be decreased.
    c. The exposure time does not matter.
    d. none of the above

CHAPTER APPLICATION

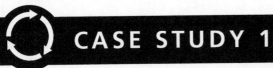

CASE STUDY 1

In the course of the day, the dental assistant has obtained images on adults and children and for special requests. Each of these assignments required choosing a particular film type.

1. A full mouth series was required for an adult. What intraoral image receptor size would typically be used?

   _____

   _____

2. In this adult case, there is severe crowding in the anterior. What size image receptor might be necessary?

   _____

   _____

3. The dentist has requested an adult set of bitewings but wants only two films. The area to be covered by a No. 2 film would not be adequate. What image receptor size would be used?

   _____

   _____

4. A 4 year old patient is in need of radiographs patient. The dentist has ordered one image of the maxilla and the mandible. What image type and image receptor size would be required?

   _____

   _____

CASE STUDY 2

Holly is being examined to determine the diagnosis for recurrent caries. The dentist prescribes x-rays. Holly expresses her concerns about radiation and its effects. The dentist and the dental assistant understand that Holly needs assurance about the effects of dental x-rays compared to other radiation sources.

1. Define ALARA.

   _____

   _____

   _____

   _____

   _____

2. Define MPD.

_____

_____

_____

_____

_____

Critical Thinking

1. Knowing the composition of the intraoral film packet is necessary in order to identify its contents during film exposure and processing. Name the film packet contents.

_____

_____

_____

_____

2. The dental assistant has the responsibility to know and understand intraoral dental x-ray film types. The dentist may use one of three choices based on film speed and exposure benefits. Name the three choices normally found in the dental office, their speed differentials, and which involves the least radiation exposure for the patient.

_____

_____

_____

_____

3. Assume that a patient is to have an 18-film series (full mouth). Two methods of exposure include using a long, round PID or using a rectangular PID. Explain both methods, and identify which benefits the patient the most in terms of reduced radiation exposure.

_____

_____

_____

_____

CHAPTER **28**

Dental Radiography Infection Control, Exposure, Processing and Evaluation of Dental Radiographs, and Mounting of Radiographs

SPECIFIC INSTRUCTIONAL OBJECTIVES

At the completion of this chapter, you will be able to meet these objectives:

1. Use terms presented in this lesson.
2. Discuss the infection control protocol related to dental radiography.
3. Compare and contrast the sequence of exposures in the bisecting technique and the paralleling technique.
4. Compare and contrast patient position during the bisecting technique and the paralleling technique.
5. Compare and contrast the image receptor holders in the bisecting technique and the paralleling technique.
6. Discuss image receptor placement for bitewing images.
7. Discuss image receptor placement for periapical images.
8. Discuss the importance of angulation during intraoral exposures.
9. State the cause of a conecut image.
10. Explain the errors caused by image receptor placement.
11. Differentiate between elongation and foreshortening.
12. Discuss interproximal overlap.
13. Describe the errors that may be caused during exposure.

14. State the purpose of occlusal images.

15. State the procedure for exposing adult occlusal images.

16. Discuss image receptor placement during modified exposure techniques.

17. List the steps in exposing a pediatric full set of images.

18. Explain the protocol for management of patients with special needs.

19. Discuss the protocol for maintaining radiographic records.

20. Compare and contrast the developer and fixer solutions.

21. Compare and contrast the manual processing technique and the autoprocessing technique.

22. Describe the components of the darkroom.

23. Describe the manual processing tank.

24. Explain the importance of checking the temperature of the manual processing solutions.

25. Outline the steps in the manual processing technique.

26. Outline the steps in the automatic processing technique.

27. Compare and contrast solutions for automatic processors and manual processors.

28. Discuss the maintenance of processing equipment.

29. Identify film processing errors.

30. Outline the steps in mounting traditional films.

31. Compare and contrast the lingual mounting view and the labial mounting view.

32. State the sequence of viewing mounted radiographs in a full mouth series.

33. Outline the steps in film duplication.

VOCABULARY BUILDER

Matching

Match each term with the appropriate definition.

1. _____ gutta percha
2. _____ bisecting the angle technique
3. _____ Cieszynski's Rule of Isometry
4. _____ conecut
5. _____ herringbone pattern
6. _____ topographical projection
7. _____ cross-sectional

a. items such as glasses that may appear on a radiographic image

b. imprint of lead foil on film due to reversed film placement in XCP

c. without teeth

d. white areas on an image

e. dark areas on an image

f. hardens emulsion on film base

g. oxygen causing darkening of chemical

8. _____ edentulous

9. _____ selective reduction

10. _____ fixer

11. _____ radiopaque

12. _____ radiolucent

13. _____ oxidation

14. _____ fogged film

15. _____ reticulation

16. _____ labial mounting

17. _____ artifact

18. _____ horizontal angulation

h. grayish appearance of film

i. provides view of anterior of palate

j. also known as right angle projection

k. error caused by receptor not centered in XCP ring

l. silver halide crystals converted to black metal silver

m. root canal filling material

n. method used for dental radiographic exposures

o. geometric rule

p. preferred method for placing films in holder

q. appearance of cracked film emulsion

r. side to side movement of PID

CHAPTER REVIEW

Multiple Choice

1. Which of the following is correct regarding the types of instruments used in dental radiography?

   a. Image receptor holders such as XCP kits are considered semicritical instruments and must be sterilized prior to reuse on another patient.

   b. Surfaces that may be contaminated during dental radiology procedures are considered to be critical instruments and should be disinfected and/or covered with a barrier.

   c. The dental x-ray machine head is considered to be a critical instrument which may be contaminated and should be covered with a barrier and/or disinfected.

   d. The digital sensor is considered to be a critical instrument and should be sterilized for use on each patient.

2. Which of the following is the correct sequence for exposing a full mouth series using size 2 image receptors with the paralleling technique?

   a. maxillary right canine, maxillary incisors, maxillary left canine, mandibular left canine, mandibular incisors, mandibular right canine, maxillary right premolars, maxillary right molars, mandibular left premolars, mandibular left molars, maxillary left premolars, maxillary left molars, mandibular right premolars, mandibular right molars

   b. maxillary right canine, maxillary incisors, maxillary left canine, mandibular right canine, mandibular incisors, mandibular left canine, maxillary right premolars, maxillary right molars, mandibular left premolars, mandibular left molars, maxillary left premolars, maxillary left molars, mandibular right premolars, mandibular right molars

   c. maxillary right canine, maxillary incisors, maxillary left canine, mandibular left canine, mandibular incisors, mandibular right canine, maxillary left premolars, maxillary left molars, maxillary right premolars, maxillary right molars, mandibular left premolars, mandibular left molars, mandibular right premolars, mandibular right molars

   d. maxillary right canine, maxillary incisors, maxillary left canine, mandibular left canine, mandibular incisors, mandibular right canine, maxillary right premolars, maxillary right molars, mandibular right premolars, mandibular right molars, maxillary left premolars, maxillary left molars, mandibular left premolars, mandibular left molars

3. Which of the following holders is not used to obtain images during the bisecting technique?

   a. Snap-A-Ray holders

   b. disposable bit blocks

   c. patient's finger to stabilize receptor

   d. loop type tabs for bitewings

4. When obtaining the molar bitewing image, the image receptor should be centered on the premolars. The front edge of the receptor should be aligned with the midline of the second premolar in order to obtain the first and second molars centered in the image.

   Select the correct response based on the statements above

   a. Both statements are true.

   b. Both statements are false.

   c. The first statement is true; the second statement is false.

   d. The first statement is false; the second statement is true.

5. Horizontal angulation should be zero for bitewing exposures. If the horizontal angle is not zero, the beam does not go directly through the contacts between the teeth and overlap may occur.

   Select the correct response based on the statement above

   a. Both statements are true.

   b. Both statements are false.

   c. The first statement is true; the second statement is false.

   d. The first statement is false; the second statement is true.

6. Which of the following image receptor placement error occurs when the traditional film is placed reverse in the oral cavity?

   a. elongation

   b. conecut

   c. herring bone

   d. dot of film at apex

7. Which of the following is not correct regarding placement of the mandibular occlusal cross-sectional projection?

   a. The traditional size 4 film is placed with white side of film toward the mandible.

   b. The image receptor is placed long from side to side with just ¼ inch beyond the labial of incisors.

   c. The PID is set with the central ray at 65 degrees to the image receptor.

   d. The patient is positioned supine, and the patient's head is tilted back so the mandible is perpendicular to the floor.

8. Which of the following is correct regarding the pediatric mandibular cross-sectional occlusal projection?

   a. The maxilla should be parallel to the floor.

   b. The center of the chin is centered in the position indicating device (PID).

   c. The central ray (CR) comes in at a 45-degree angle to the image receptor.

   d. The patient is positioned upright for this exposure.

9. Which of the following is not correct when managing a patient with special needs during radiographic exposures?

   a. Advance preparation of the treatment area and supplies will help make the procedure go more smoothly.

   b. Work as slowly as possible so the patient is comfortable.

   c. A parent or guardian may need to assist during radiographic exposures.

   d. Speak with the caregiver to gain an understanding of how best to accommodate the patient's needs.

10. Which of the following is correct regarding the developing solution?

    a. The developing solution produces the radiopaque areas on an image through selective reduction.
    b. Crystals that do not receive any x-radiation are unchanged by the developer.
    c. Hydroquinone is the reducing agent in the developer.
    d. Sodium sulfite is the preservative in the developer.

11. Which of the following is not correct regarding autoprocessing?

    a. Autoprocessors do not have a water rinse step between developing and fixing of films.
    b. The solutions used by autoprocessors are not the same as those used for manual processors.
    c. The autoprocessors are able to process films more quickly because the solutions are heated to high temperatures.
    d. The autoprocessor solutions may be used in a manual processing tank if needed.

12. Which of the following is correct regarding the darkroom safelight?

    a. It should be a 7 to 15 watt bulb that allows the red-orange spectrum to come through.
    b. It should be at least 4 feet away from the workspace where films are processed.
    c. Exposure of the films to the safelight for more than 3 minutes may cause the image to disappear.
    d. Films should be exposed to the safelight for no more than 3 minutes.

13. Which of the following is not correct regarding maintenance of manual processing tanks and equipment?

    a. The hangers used for manual processing should be cleaned regularly as the residual chemicals may affect the quality of the films.
    b. The work area for processing of films should be disinfected and cleaned to ensure no residual solutions will affect the quality of films.
    c. When the solutions need to be replaced, the insert tanks should be cleaned, washed, and dried before filling with new solutions.
    d. The master tank, since it contains only water, does not need to be cleaned.

14. What is the correct sequence of steps in film mounting after gathering of all supplies and washing hands? Put each item below in number order.

    a. Place the bitewing radiographs in the mount with premolars toward the center of the mount and molars toward the outside of the mount.
    b. Label mount with patient's name, date of exposure, operator's name and dentist's name.
    c. Turn on viewbox.
    d. Place the posterior periapical radiographs. The molars should be placed toward the outside, and the bicuspids (premolars) toward the inside.
    e. Categorize all radiographs into three groups: bitewings, anterior, and posterior.
    f. Put the anterior radiographs in place, with the maxillary images above and the mandibular images below and central incisor images in the middle.

15. Which of the following is correct regarding mounting views?

    a. The lingual mounting view is the preferred method of mounting radiographs.
    b. The labial mounting view is viewed as if the dentist is seeing the patient from the front of the face.
    c. In the lingual mounting method, the convex side of the dot faces the viewer.
    d. The lingual mounting method is the approved method of the American Dental Association.

16. What is the correct sequence of steps in film duplication under darkroom safelight conditions? Put the following steps in order.

    a. Close the duplicator and press start.

    b. Position the film on the duplicating machine with convex side of dot facing up.

    c. Process film in darkroom either in tanks or in an autoprocessor and label.

    d. Remove duplicating film from box and place emulsion side down, the notch on film should be in upper right corner of duplicating machine.

Matching

Match the following darkroom equipment with the correct description of its functions.

1. _____ timer

    a. used to mix the developer and the fixer to ensure uniformity of the solutions

2. _____ thermometer

    b. used to clip films for placing in the developer and fixer tanks and the water bath

3. _____ stirring rods

    c. used to ensure that the films are in the developer and fixer for the appropriate amount of time as determined by the time-temperature chart

4. _____ film hangers

    d. used to measure the temperature of the developer and determine how long films should be in the developer

5. _____ drying racks

    e. used for drying of films after processing has been completed

CERTIFICATION REVIEW

Multiple Choice

1. What is the acceptable method of infection control for phosphor storage plates during radiographic exposures?

    a. autoclave

    b. high-level disinfectant

    c. barrier sleeves

    d. infection control not necessary

2. What is the best way to prevent cross-contamination of the control panel of the dental radiology machine?

    a. Place it in the autoclave after each patient.

    b. Use barriers.

    c. Spray it liberally with an approved disinfectant.

    d. Wipe with alcohol soaked gauze.

3. On a bitewing radiograph, you notice that one tooth is superimposed over the one next to it. What is this called?

    a. reticulation

    b. conecut

    c. overlap

    d. tilted occlusal plane

4. Why should processed films be handled by the edges?

    a. to prevent reticulation

    b. to prevent foreshortening

    c. to prevent elongation

    d. to prevent contamination

5. You notice that one of the processed films has two distinct images on it. What may have caused this error?

    a. One film was exposed twice.

    b. The film was overprocessed.

    c. The film was underprocessed.

    d. Two exposed films got stuck together in the processor.

6. You will be exposing an adult full mouth series with a size 2 image receptor. How many anterior images will you be taking?

    a. 7

    b. 6

    c. 8

    d. 5

7. What is the purpose of horizontal bitewing images?

    a. to evaluate for occlusal decay

    b. to evaluate for root decay

    c. to evaluate for interproximal decay

    d. to evaluate for periodontal disease

8. What will be the appearance of an overexposed film?

    a. light

    b. dark

    c. will have white spots

    d. will have dark spots

9. You will be taking adult occlusal images on an edentulous patient. What size image receptor should you use?

    a. 0

    b. 1

    c. 2

    d. 4

10. You will be taking a full set of radiographs on a patient who is a gagger. How should you manage this patient?

    a. Work silently so the patient does not get anxious.

    b. Tell the patient they are imagining the gagging.

    c. Use distraction techniques during the exposures.

    d. Discuss gagging in detail with the patient.

CHAPTER APPLICATION

CASE STUDY 1

During Vernon's 12-month dental exam, the dentist prescribes routine bitewings. Taken correctly, bitewing images can be used for diagnosing teeth and the surrounding structures.

1. What specific areas do bitewing radiographs show?

_____

_____

2. Bitewing radiographs are also known as

_____

_____

3. Bitewings are exposed in which areas of the oral cavity?

_____

_____

4. What specifically is detected on bitewing images?

_____

_____

5. Describe the differences between horizontal and vertical bitewings.

_____

_____

CASE STUDY 2

At 7-year-old Scott's routine dental exam, the dentist observes new decay and loose teeth. The dentist prescribes a full-mouth series of radiographs to help in determining Scott's present dental health.

1. What will a full-mouth series detect?

_____

_____

2. Will the number of films taken for Scott be the same as for an adult?

_____

_____

3. Is radiation exposure time the same for children and adults?

_____

_____

CASE STUDY 3

Dental assistant Ella has taken her first full-mouth series of radiographs using traditional films. The films are dry, and she begins to mount them.

1. What equipment and supplies are required for mounting radiographs?

_____

_____

2. What information is necessary for labeling the mount, and will it be entered in pen or in pencil?

_____

_____

3. What direction should the dot on the film face? What is this called?

_____

_____

4. What mounting technique is used in most dental offices and is recommended by the ADA?

_____

_____

5. In mounting a full-mouth set of radiographs, dividing them into three groups is recommended. Name the three groups.

_____

_____

Critical Thinking

1. Taking radiographs is part of a routine dental exam. How frequently are bitewing images taken? What specific features are detected in these x-rays?

_____

_____

_____

2. There are two methods used to mount a full series of x-rays. State the name of each method and explain the difference between the two.

_____

_____

_____

Extraoral Radiography, Digital Radiography, and Radiographic Interpretation

SPECIFIC INSTRUCTIONAL OBJECTIVES

At the completion of this chapter, you will be able to meet these objectives:

1. Use terms presented in this chapter.
2. State the purpose of extraoral radiographs.
3. Discuss panoramic radiography.
4. Describe the panoramic machine.
5. List the steps in a patient panoramic exposure.
6. Compare and contrast common panoramic radiographic errors.
7. Discuss other extraoral images used in dentistry.
8. Compare and contrast digital radiography and traditional film-based radiography.
9. Differentiate between indirect digital and direct digital dental radiography.
10. Compare and contrast the advantages and disadvantages of digital radiography.
11. List the steps in obtaining intraoral digital dental images.
12. Discuss three-dimensional imaging in dentistry.
13. Discuss the benefits of hand-held intraoral radiology units.
14. Identify the normal anatomical structures on a dental radiograph.
15. Identify dental pathologies on a radiographic image.
16. Identify periodontal pathologies on a radiographic image.

17. Discuss dental anomalies that may be seen on a dental radiograph.

18. Identify commonly used dental materials as they appear on a dental radiograph.

19. Discuss quality management protocol related to dental radiology.

20. Discuss the laws related to dental radiology.

21. State the responsibilities of the dental assistant as the radiographer.

22. Discuss the steps in risk management.

23. Discuss the relationship of HIPAA to dental radiographs.

VOCABULARY BUILDER

Matching

Match each term with the appropriate definition.

1. _____ tomography

2. _____ rotational centers

3. _____ intensifying screens

4. _____ rare earth phosphors

5. _____ calcium tungstate phosphors

6. _____ analog

7. _____ pixel

8. _____ charge couple device

9. _____ photostimulable phosphor

10. _____ cone beam computed tomography

11. _____ axial

12. _____ sagittal

13. _____ coronal

14. _____ respondeat superior

15. _____ condensing osteitis

a. type of image produced by x-rays striking traditional film

b. means "part"

c. type of technology used in digital sensor

d. view from below chin to top of head

e. view from behind head to front of face

f. indirect digital imaging

g. side to side view

h. axis around which panoramic tubehead rotates

i. emits blue light

j. pieces of a digital image

k. emits green light

l. radiopaque area around tooth apex

m. let the superior reply

n. three-dimensional imaging

o. line the panoramic cassette

CHAPTER REVIEW

Matching

Match each component of the panoramic unit with its function.

Component

1. _____ exposure controls
2. _____ head positioner
3. _____ x-ray tubehead
4. _____ cassette

Function

a. flat, hard container that holds the film

b. collimator has narrow vertical slit

c. outside the x-ray room; includes kV and mA

d. chin rest, notched bite-block, and forehead rest

Match the American Association of Periodontology stages of periodontal disease with the correct description.

1. _____ Stage I mild periodontitis

2. _____ Stage II moderate periodontitis

3. _____ Stage III advanced periodontitis

4. _____ Stage IV severe periodontitis

a. bone loss from middle 1/3 of tooth and beyond; greater than five missing teeth

b. bone loss from middle 1/3 of tooth and beyond; less than four missing teeth

c. less than 15% bone loss at the coronal 1/3; no missing teeth

d. 15 to 33% bone loss at the coronal 1/3; no missing teeth

Match the dental pathology description with the correct name.

1. _____ Decay appears as a triangle in the enamel; visible on radiograph but present only in enamel and less than halfway through the enamel

2. _____ Decay not visible on radiograph; clinical exam reveals dark pits and fissures, which may be sticky

3. _____ Occurs on the cementum of teeth and appears as a saucer shaped radiolucency on images

4. _____ Decay not visible on radiographs; decay is more than halfway through enamel but has not yet reached the dentinoenamel junction (DEJ)

5. _____ Decay visible on radiographs but present only in enamel and more than halfway through the enamel; decay has not yet reached the DEJ

6. _____ Occurs under an existing restoration

7. _____ Decay is visible on radiograph as an oval shaped radiolucency under the occlusal enamel and has entered dentin; decay is less than halfway through dentin toward pulp

8. _____ Decay is visible on radiograph and has entered dentin; decay appears as a second triangle in the dentin; the first triangle is in the enamel; decay is less than halfway through dentin toward pulp

9. _____ Decay appears as a large radiolucency under the occlusal surface of the tooth and is more than halfway toward the pulp

10. _____ Decay appears as a large radiolucency in the interproximal area and is more than halfway toward the pulp

11. _____ Occurs on buccal and lingual surfaces of teeth; a clinical exam is needed to determine location

12. _____ Decay present on multiple teeth throughout oral cavity

13. _____ Appears as a radiopaque dense bone that develops periapically in response to chronic pulpal involvement or necrosis

14. _____ Resorption that occurs within the pulp tissue of the tooth

15. _____ Infection that develops at the apex of the tooth and appears as a radiolucency

16. _____ Resorption starts on the outside surface of a tooth and progresses inward

17. _____ Calcified structures that appear as radiopacities in the pulp of the tooth

18. _____ Root resorption occurs during normal exfoliation due to the pressure of the erupting tooth

19. _____ Visible on a radiograph as a wider radiolucent area around the root of the tooth

    a. incipient occlusal decay
    b. incipient interproximal decay
    c. moderate occlusal decay
    d. moderate interproximal decay
    e. advanced occlusal decay
    f. advanced interproximal decay
    g. severe occlusal decay
    h. severe interproximal decay
    i. recurrent decay
    j. rampant decay
    k. smooth surface decay
    l. root decay
    m. widened periodontal ligament space
    n. pulp stones
    o. periapical abscess
    p. condensing osteitis
    q. internal resorption
    r. external resorption
    s. physiological resorption

Multiple Choice

1. Which of the following may be identified by extraoral radiographs?

    a. large areas of the skull on a single radiograph
    b. both maxillary and mandibular areas at the same time
    c. conditions or artifacts that are not otherwise diagnosed in other ways
    d. all of the above

2. Panoramic radiographs may be taken on which of the following patients?

    a. patients who have trismus
    b. patients in wheelchairs
    c. edentulous patients
    d. all of the above

3. Which of the following is not an extraoral radiograph?

a. panoramic

b. periapical

c. cephalometric

d. transcranial temporomandibular joint

CERTIFICATION REVIEW

Multiple Choice

1. After you process films in the darkroom, you notice the films are fogged. Which test would you perform if you believe it is the safelight that may be causing the film fog?

a. kVp

b. mA

c. coin test

d. stepwedge

2. How often should the developing solution be tested with the use of a stepwedge?

a. annually

b. every 6 months

c. monthly

d. daily

3. Which term describes the compact edge of the cortical bone that shows as a radiopaque point between the teeth when visualized on a radiograph?

a. genial tubercle

b. mandibular canal

c. coronoid process

d. alveolar crest

4. What is the appearance of metallic restorations on a radiographic image?

a. radiopaque

b. radiolucent

c. either A or B

d. neither A or B

5. What positioning error has occurred when taking a panoramic radiograph if the anterior teeth appear blurred and the spine appears superimposed over the ramus areas of the mandible?

a. Patient is positioned too far back.

b. Patient's head is tilted downward.

c. Patient's head is tilted upward.

d. Patient is positioned too far forward.

6. Which of the following will not cause a ghost image?

a. an earring

b. eyeglasses

c. caries

d. a facial piercing

7. What positioning error has occurred when taking a panoramic radiograph if a dark radiolucent area appears above the apices of the maxillary teeth?

    a. Patient is positioned too far back.

    b. Patient's tongue was not resting on the roof of the mouth.

    c. Patient's head is tilted upward.

    d. Patient is positioned too far forward.

8. When taking a panoramic radiograph, the line from the tragus of the ear to the floor of the obit should be parallel to the floor. What is this line called?

    a. midsagittal plane

    b. lateral

    c. transcranial

    d. Frankfort plane

9. On a radiograph, which term describes the radiolucent area on the lingual side of the mandible at the midline?

    a. lamina dura

    b. mental foramen

    c. lingual foramen

    d. mandibular foramen

10. What is the type of imaging most often used when planning an implant surgery?

    a. panoramic imaging

    b. cone beam computed tomography

    c. magnetic resonance imaging

    d. cephalometric imaging

CHAPTER APPLICATION

CASE STUDY

Dental assistant Katie is preparing to interpret radiographs. Being familiar with the terminology used in radiographic interpretation and learning landmarks will make this step easier and more meaningful.

1. Define landmarks.

    _____

    _____

    _____

2. Identify each of the following as radiopaque or radiolucent: enamel, dentin, cementum, pulp chamber, pulp canals, periodontal ligament, lamina dura, cortical plate, cancellous bone, and cortical bone.

    _____

    _____

    _____

⊠ **Critical Thinking**

1. What causes a lead apron artifact in a panoramic radiograph?

   _____

   _____

2. Each manufacturer of digital radiography equipment provides detailed instructions on preparation of the equipment and computer. Name two advantages and two disadvantages of digital radiography.

   _____

   _____

3. Describe the advantages of three-dimensional radiography.

   _____

   _____

   _____

   _____

4. As the dental assistant it is your job to maintain quality assurance of the darkroom. You decide to test for film fog. Upon processing of the film that had the coin on it under safelight condition, you notice that the film emerged with the image of the coin. What is your next step to determine the cause of the film fog?

   _____

   _____

   _____

   _____

5. What are the steps to take for risk management related to dental radiography?

   _____

   _____

   _____

   _____

   _____

   _____

   _____

   _____

6. List the correct sequence of steps for intraoral digital exposures using a direct digital imaging system.

   _____

   _____

Assist with Restorative Procedures and Dental Materials

CHAPTER 30

Dental Emergency Procedures and Dental Cements

SPECIFIC INSTRUCTIONAL OBJECTIVES

At the completion of this chapter, you will be able to meet these objectives:

1. Use the terms presented in this chapter.
2. Discuss emergency treatment for soft tissue oral trauma.
3. Recall the cause and emergency treatment for oral lesions.
4. Describe the appearance and treatment of periodontal tissue injuries.
5. Differentiate between classifications of tooth fractures.
6. Recall signs, symptoms, and treatment of the progression of dental caries.
7. Describe cavity preparation form and structure.
8. State the guidelines for mixing dental cements.
9. Describe the use, composition, properties, and manipulation considerations of dental cements.
10. Describe the steps in preparing for and placing temporary cement restorations.

VOCABULARY BUILDER

Matching

Match each term with the appropriate definition.

1. _____ homo-
2. _____ –eous
3. _____ necro-
4. _____ ankyl-
5. _____ avulse
6. _____ cavo-
7. _____ palliate

a. to grow together
b. to lesson severity of pain
c. composed of
d. tear away forcibly
e. dead tissue
f. cavity
g. same

8. _____ margin   a. remove tissue by scraping

9. _____ base   b. violent fall injury

10. _____ concuss   c. passage formed by disease

11. _____ contuse   d. a border

12. _____ curettage   e. cements objects together

13. _____ erode   f. bottom layer

14. _____ fistula   g. injury without breaking the skin

15. _____ luting   h. eat into

Fill in the Blank

Please fill in the blank with one of the choices provided.

stropping   cavosurface margin   axial wall

cavity preparation   cavity preparation

1. The _____ is the internal internal long axis of the tooth in the cavity preparation.

2. _____ is when the mixing technique uses a back and forth pressing motion.

3. The process of removing caries and unsupported tooth structures is called _____.

4. The remaining tooth structure shaped to support a dental restoration is called the _____.

5. The _____ is the exterior surface of the tooth's cavity preparation.

CHAPTER REVIEW

True or False

Circle whether the answer is true or false.

1. **T   F**   Zinc phosphate cement has reached the luting consistency when the material is creamy and follows the spatula about 1 inch above the mixing slab.

2. **T   F**   Reinforced zinc oxide–eugenol cement used as temporary restoration has a putty-like consistency and rolls on the mixing slab.

3. **T   F**   Bases are applied between the tooth and the restoration to protect the pulp.

4. **T   F**   When dispensing a two-paste zinc oxide–eugenol cement, the accelerator should be half the length of the base.

5. A plastic filling instrument is used to place the dental cement into the cavity preparation. The amalgam condenser presses it against the floor of the preparation.

   a. Both statements are true.

   b. Both statements are false.

   c. The first statement is true; the second statement is false.

   d. The first statement is false; the second statement is true.

Matching

Match the dental cement to its primary use.

1. _____ zinc oxide–eugenol

2. _____ reinforced zinc oxide–eugenol

3. _____ glass ionomer

4. _____ resin cement

5. _____ resin-modified glass ionomer

a. cement porcelain-fused-to-metal restoration

b. cement ceramic indirect restoration

c. palliative base

d. temporary restoration

e. cement orthodontic bands and brackets

Multiple Choice

1. When would an insulating base be used?

    1. when a tooth has a large amount of dentin removed
    2. when there is danger of thermal sensitivity from a restoration
    3. when there is a shallow cavity preparation
    4. before all indirect restorations
        a. 1, 2
        b. 2, 3
        c. 4
        d. 1, 2, 4

2. Which cement(s) are used when cementing a temporary indirect restoration?

    a. zinc oxide–eugenol cement
    b. polycarboxylate cement
    c. zinc phosphate cement
    d. glass ionomer

3. When would luting agents be used?

    1. to soothe and promote healing in trauma situations
    2. to cement crowns and bridges in place
    3. to cement orthodontic appliances in place
    4. when there is a fracture or deep caries
        a. 1, 2, 3
        b. 2, 3
        c. 3
        d. 1, 2, 3, 4

4. Because of the exothermic properties of zinc phosphate, it is generally mixed slowly in increments

    a. with a plastic instrument.
    b. on a paper mixing pad.
    c. on a cool glass slab.
    d. in a dappen dish.

5. What ingredient in zinc oxide–eugenol soothes tooth structures?

    a. fluoride
    b. clove oil
    c. calcium
    d. phosphorus

6. Which dental cement is the best choice for a temporary restoration for pulpitis due to it sedative properties?

    a. zinc oxide–eugenol cement
    b. polycarboxylate cement
    c. IRM
    d. glass ionomer

7. Which dental cement is it appropriate to mix on a paper mixing pad?

    1. zinc phosphate
    2. zinc oxide–eugenol

3. polycarboxylate

4. glass ionomer

    a. 1, 4

    b. 1, 2, 3

    c. 1, 3, 4

    d. 2, 3, 4

8. Which dental cement is most often used as an intermediate restorative material?

    a. resin

    b. zinc phosphate

    c. glass ionomer

    d. zinc oxide–eugenol

9. What kind of dental caries does fluoride-releasing restorative materials help to prevent?

    a. rampant

    b. recurrent

    c. incipient

    d. root

10. The process of mixing cements to its primary consistency is known as

    a. luting.

    b. desiccation.

    c. wetting.

    d. lining.

CERTIFICATION REVIEW

Multiple Choice

1. In which dental emergency does the patient present with constant pain that worsens when they lay down?

    a. reversible pulpitis

    b. irreversible pulpitis

    c. acute pulpitis

    d. chronic periapical abscess

2. Which treatment is recommended for an avulsed tooth?

    a. rinsing the tooth in warm water

    b. scrubbing the tooth with antiseptic wipe

    c. replanting the tooth quickly

    d. there is no successful treatment

3. A tooth that is partially dislocated and has increased mobility due to trauma or injury is said to be

    a. avulsed.

    b. subluxated.

    c. intruded.

    d. extruded.

4. When would zinc phosphate cement be used in operative dentistry?

    a. cementing temporary crowns

    b. in place of a cavity liner

    c. when cementing permanent restorations

    d. as a soothing base

5. When would polycarboxylate cement be used?

   a. as a base

   b. as a liner

   c. to cement temporary restorations

   d. as a core buildup material

6. When would zinc oxide–eugenol be used?

   a. as a liner

   b. as base under composite restorations

   c. as an insulating base material

   d. as a permanent cement

7. What is released slowly into tooth structures from a glass ionomer?

   a. phosphoric acid

   b. calcium

   c. clove oil

   d. fluoride

8. Which material is used as a pulp-capping material?

   a. glass ionomer

   b. zinc phosphate

   c. zinc oxide–eugenol

   d. polycarboxylate cement

9. Which cement is recommended to be mixed on a cool, dry glass slab?

   a. glass ionomer

   b. zinc phosphate

   c. zinc oxide–eugenol

   d. polycarboxylate

10. Which cement has an exothermic reaction during mixing?

   a. glass ionomer

   b. zinc phosphate

   c. calcium hydroxide

   d. polycarboxylate

CHAPTER APPLICATION

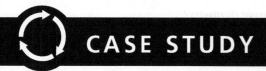

CASE STUDY

Damon called the dental office complaining that he fell while skateboarding and fractured his two front teeth. The reception scheduled him for an immediate emergency appointment. After taking radiographs and an oral examination, the dentist asks the assistant to note a tooth 8 enamel and dentin fracture without a pulp exposure and a 9 fracture involving the enamel, dentin, and pulp.

1. Using the Ellis tooth fracture classification, what classification should be noted in the chart of tooth 8?

_____

2. Using the Ellis tooth fracture classification, what classification should be noted in the chart of tooth 9?

_____

3. What emergency treatment should be performed on tooth 8?

_____

4. What emergency treatment should be performed on tooth 9?

_____

5. What follow-up treatment should be scheduled for tooth 9?

_____

Image Labeling

Name the following labeled line angles

1. _____ What line angle is labeled as #1?

2. _____ What line angle is labeled as #2?

3. _____ What line angle is labeled as #3?

4. _____ What line angle is labeled as #7?

5. _____ What line angle is labeled as #8?

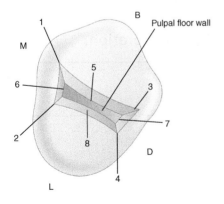

FIGURE 30-1

Cavity preparation line angles
(looking down on an occlusal
view).

CHAPTER 31

Amalgam Procedure and Materials

SPECIFIC INSTRUCTIONAL OBJECTIVES

At the completion of this chapter, you will be able to meet these objectives:

1. Use terms presented in this chapter.

2. Discuss dental material properties.

3. Recall agencies and organizations regulating dental materials.

4. Describe treatment of cavity preparation for placement of dental amalgam.

5. Identify the different matrix band systems and their uses.

6. List advantages and disadvantages in using dental amalgam as a direct restoration.

7. Explain the clinical importance of the properties of amalgam.

8. Discuss mercury hygiene for patients and for dental workers.

9. Describe the steps in completing an amalgam restoration.

10. Discuss the indications and contraindications for finishing and polishing amalgam restorations.

11. Describe the steps in finishing and polishing an amalgam restoration.

VOCABULARY BUILDER

Matching

Match each term with the appropriate definition.

1. _____ alloy

2. _____ flush

3. _____ therm

4. _____ solvent

5. _____ sphere

a. heat

b. ball shaped

c. even with surface

d. mixture of metals

e. substance dissolved by another

6. _____ ductility   a. triangular shape

7. _____ esthetic   b. discoloration of metal surface

8. _____ finish   c. smooth a surface

9. _____ tarnish   d. concerned with appearance

10. _____ wedge   e. ability to be hammered or stretched without breaking

Multiple Choice

1. _____ is the process of combining metal alloys and mercury.

   a. Comminutation

   b. Malleability

   c. Retention

   d. Amalgamation

2. Improper carving or finishing an amalgam can cause concave areas at the margins of the restoration referred to as _____.

   a. flash

   b. flush

   c. ditching

   d. open margin

3. When the dentist requests that the material be _____, the alloy and mercury are mixed in a capsule.

   a. polished

   b. finished

   c. triturated

   d. pulverised

4. A material is _____ when it can be shaped by pressing without breaking.

   a. retentive

   b. malleable

   c. ductile

   d. impervious

5. _____ occurs when excess amalgam leaks out of the matrix band.

   a. Overhang

   b. Flush

   c. Ditching

   d. Open margin

6. _____ is the seepage of saliva and debris from the oral cavity between the tooth structure and the restorative materials.

   a. Flow

   b. Ductility

   c. Malleability

   d. Microleakage

7. _____ is the ability of a material to transmit heat.

   a. Dimensional change

   b. Microleakage

   c. Thermal conductivity

   d. Stress and strain

8. _____ is the result of chemical or electrochemical attacks on pure metal in the oral environment, causing deep pitting and roughness.

   a. Tarnishing

   b. Corrosion

   c. Shearing

   d. Ductility

9. _____ is a combination of an alloy and mercury.

   a. Composite

   b. Amalgam

   c. Glass ionomer

   d. Resin

10. A _____ is used in finishing the interproximals of the amalgam restoration.

   a. finishing bur

   b. finishing strip

   c. finishing stone

   d. all of these

CHAPTER REVIEW

True or False

Circle whether the answer is true or false.

1. **T   F**   Stones are used when adjusting or polishing an amalgam restoration.

2. **T   F**   A cavity varnish is used to seal the dentinal tubules of the cavity preparation.

3. **T   F**   The base of a wedge is placed toward the occlusal surface.

4. **T   F**   An example of shearing stress and strain is bruxism, or grinding of the teeth.

5. **T   F**   Flow, or creep and slump, is the continuous deformation of a solid.

Matching

Match each term with the appropriate definition.

1. _____ calcium hydroxide

2. _____ cavity varnish

3. _____ carver

4. _____ burnisher

5. _____ condenser

6. _____ amalgam carrier

a. used to smooth condensed amalgam

b. stimulates reparative dentin

c. used to transport amalgam to cavity preparation

d. used to shape condensed amalgam

e. used to press amalgam into cavity preparation

f. seals dentin tubules

Multiple Choice

1. What is the purpose of using amalgam bonding agents?

   a. increases retention of amalgam restoration

   b. decreases microleakage

   c. allow for a more conservation amalgam restoration

   d. all of these

2. Which phrases describe dental amalgam?

   1. primarily used for posterior restorations
   2. economical restoration
   3. will last several year
   4. triturated with alloy materials and mercury

   a. 1, 3

   b. 2, 4

   c. 2, 3

   d. 1, 2, 3, 4

3. All of the following are true about mercury EXCEPT that

a. it is metal in a liquid state.

b. it is not toxic.

c. vaporizes at low room temperature.

d. scraps should be kept in sealed container.

4. Which metals are in the composition of dental amalgam alloy?

a. silver, tin, copper, and aluminum

b. silver, tin, zinc, and gold

c. silver, tin, copper, and zinc

d. tin, zinc, mercury, and copper

5. Which part of the universal (Tofflemire) matrix retainer holds the ends of the matrix band in place in the diagonal slot?

a. spindle

b. vise

c. guide channels

d. inner knob

6. The sectional matrix system benefits tooth contour by

a. restoring anatomic contacts.

b. acting as a stabilizing matrix.

c. producing a tight contact.

d. all of the above

7. The occlusal edge of the Tofflemire matrix band should extend no more than _____ mm above the highest cusp.

a. 1

b. 1.5

c. 2

d. 2.5

8. Which part of the universal (Tofflemire) matrix retainer adjust the size of the matrix band loop?

a. spindle

b. outer knob

c. guide channels

d. inner knob

9. To ensure contact with the adjacent tooth, the Tofflemire matrix band

a. needs to be straight.

b. requires contouring with a burnisher.

c. must be concave at the contact area.

d. needs to be held by a wedge.

CERTIFICATION REVIEW

Multiple Choice

1. When is the cavity varnish applied?

a. before the cavity liner and base material

b. after cavity liner but before base material

c. never used with base material

d. never used with a cavity liner

2. What is the next step after the amalgam filling material has been condensed into the Class II cavity preparation?

a. Place the matrix band.

b. Insert the wooden wedge.

c. Burnish the restoration.

d. Remove the dental dam.

3. Which is the correct sequence of dental instruments based on order of use for a Class I amalgam restoration tray setup?

    a. excavator, amalgam carrier, cleoid-discoid, burnisher

    b. excavator, condenser, burnisher, cleoid-discoid

    c. excavator, matrix band, amalgam carrier, cleoid-discoid, burnisher

    d. excavator, matrix band, condenser, burnisher, cleoid-discoid

4. How should a universal matrix band be removed?

    a. Lift the band from the mesial direction.

    b. Lift the band in an occlusal direction.

    c. Pull the band from the distal portion first.

    d. Pull the band toward the gingiva first.

5. Which of the following should be included on the tray setup for a Class II amalgam restoration for tooth 30?

    a. universal matrix band and wooden wedge

    b. mylar strip and plastic wedge

    c. T-band and wooden wedge

    d. international matrix band and plastic wedge

6. What instrument is used to carve the occlusal surface for an MOD amalgam on tooth 18?

    a. cleoid-discoid

    b. Hollenbeck

    c. plastic instrument

    d. low-speed handpiece

7. A 6-year-old patient is scheduled for a DO amalgam on tooth T. What matrix band should be on the tray setup?

    a. Tofflemire

    b. T-band

    c. mylar

    d. spot-welded

8. What may occur when an MOD amalgam is placed on tooth 3 and tooth 30 has an existing full gold crown?

    a. galvanism

    b. microleakage

    c. corrosion

    d. TMD

9. Which is a cavity detection method?

    1. radiographs

    2. probing with explorer

    3. special dye

    4. DIAGNOdent laser

    a. 1, 2

    b. 1, 2, 3

    c. 1, 2, 4

    d. 1, 2, 3, 4

10. When preparing a universal matrix band, what direction does the smaller circumference edge of the band face?

    a. toward the occlusal surface

    b. toward the gingiva

    c. toward the mesial

    d. toward the distal

CHAPTER APPLICATION

 CASE STUDY

Luigi calls into the office as an emergency complaining that he has pain after an amalgam was placed in tooth 30 by his previous dentist. Upon examination, the new dentist notices that tooth 31 has an existing full gold crown.

1. What is potentially the cause of this pain?

_____

_____

2. What is this chemical reaction called?

_____

_____

3. What can be done to alleviate this pain?

_____

_____

Image Labeling

The universal (Tofflemire) matrix is the most common matrix and retainer used for amalgam restorations. Label its parts.

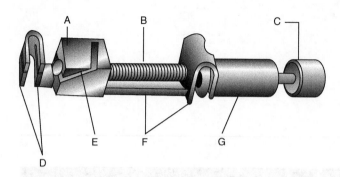

1. a. _____

2. b. _____

3. c. _____

4. d. _____

5. e. _____

6. f. _____

7. g. _____

CHAPTER 32

Composite Procedures and Materials

SPECIFIC INSTRUCTIONAL OBJECTIVES

At the completion of this chapter, you will be able to meet these objectives:

1. Use terms presented in this chapter.
2. Differentiate among the types of composite resins.
3. Explain the purpose of etching and bonding.
4. Discuss matrix systems used with composite restorations.
5. Describe the composite restoration procedure.
6. Recall the types of direct esthetic dental restorations.

VOCABULARY BUILDER

Matching

Match each term with the appropriate definition.

1. _____ com
2. _____ core
3. _____ desiccate
4. _____ etch
5. _____ filler
6. _____ smear
7. _____ prime
8. _____ veneer

a. dehydrate
b. cover with a material
c. together
d. occupies volume
e. prepare for an operation
f. innermost part
g. dissolve tooth structure
h. make dirty

9. _____ hybrid

10. _____ adhesive

11. _____ ambient

12. _____ celluloid

13. _____ chroma

14. _____ compule

15. _____ coupling

a. united by molecular force

b. clear plastic

c. color saturation

d. combination of different types of fillers

e. encircling

f. chemical joining

g. dispensing unit

Fill in the Blank

Please fill in the blank with one of the choices provided.

compomer   desiccation   hue

veneer   smear layer

1. The various shades of teeth are found on a shade guide and grouped together depending on ____ and designated by the letters A–D.

2. A small amount of moisture must remain after etching and before bonding to prevent _____ and tooth damage.

3. A _____ is the combination of a composite and glass ionomer.

4. The layer of enamel or dentin from the grinding of the dental burs during the cavity preparation is called the _____.

5. A tooth colored shell bonded to the facial of a tooth to improve the appearance is called a _____.

CHAPTER REVIEW

True or False

Circle whether the answer is true or false.

1. **T** **F** Fillers such as quartz, silica, and silicate are added to the resin composite to improve strength and wear resistance.

2. **T** **F** A coupling agent provides a bond between the fillers and the resin matrix.

3. **T** **F** Self-cured resin materials are more commonly used than light-cured resins.

4. **T** **F** When using an etchant, the patient as well as the dental team should wear protective glasses and the patient should be instructed to close their eyes.

5. **T** **F** Newer etchants do not burn the soft tissue; therefore, there is no need for special precautions to be taken.

6. **T** **F** When applying the etchant with a microbrush, the agent should be forcefully rub it onto the enamel and then dentin.

7. **T   F**   Packable composites should be cured in layers for optimum results.

8. **T   F**   A celluloid crown form is used to mold the composite for a Class IV restoration.

9. **T   F**   A retention pins may need to be placed with there is a large amount of lost tooth structure.

10. **T   F**   Self-etch bonding agent modifies instead of removing the smear layer and does not require phosphoric acid or rinsing.

Multiple Choice

1. Which material dominates the field of esthetic restorations?

   a. composite

   b. glass ionomer

   c. bonding agents

   d. polycarboxylate

2. The main component of composite restorations is which of the following?

   a. organic polymer matrix

   b. inorganic polymer particles

   c. inorganic silane matric

   d. resin silane particles

3. What types of matrix is needed when the incisal edge on anterior teeth is involved and a Class V cavity preparation on a posterior tooth is being restored with a composite restoration?

   a. sectional matrix

   b. crown-form

   c. celluloid matrix strip

   d. no matrix strip is needed

4. With which material is the plastic matrix strip used?

   a. composite

   b. glass ionomer

   c. compomer

   d. all of the above

5. This type of composite combines strength and esthetics and is used in the anterior and posterior areas of the mouth.

   a. hybrid composites

   b. microfill composites

   c. macrofill composites

   d. minifill composites

6. Which of the following holds the plastic matrix strip in place?

   a. 212 clamp

   b. Tofflemire

   c. clip retainer

   d. wedge

7. Composite restorative materials

   a. come in flowable and condensable forms.

   b. available in a variety of shades.

   c. can be light-cured, self-cured, or dual-cured.

   d. all of the above

8. Before the composite material is placed in the cavity preparation:

   a. a layer of amalgam is placed.

   b. the tooth is etched and rinsed.

   c. an enamel sealant is placed.

   d. fluoride is placed on the tooth.

9. Which type(s) of composite restorative materials have universal clinical applications and are the most popular?

1. macrofill

2. microfill

3. hybrid

4. nanofill

5. nanohybrid

    a. 1, 2   c. 3, 4

    b. 2, 3   d. 4, 5

10. After a compule of resin material has been used for the placement of a composite restoration, what should the assistant do with the compule?

    a. Wipe it using a recommended disinfecting agent.

    b. Sterilize it in dry heat oven.

    c. Wrap it in gauze soaked in intermediate disinfecting agent.

    d. Compules are single use and should be disposed of.

CERTIFICATION REVIEW

Multiple Choice

1. Which dental materials will inhibit the set of a composite restoration?

    a. calcium hydroxide liner and polycarboxylate cement

    b. glass ionomer cement and calcium hydroxide liner

    c. varnish and zinc oxide eugenol

    d. glass ionomer and polycarboxylate cement

2. Which is the sequence of use of materials for placing Class II composite restoration when both the enamel and dentin are involved?

    a. bonding agent, liner, etchant, primer

    b. primer, etchant, liner, bonding agent

    c. etchant, liner, bonding agent, primer

    d. liner, etchant, primer, bonding agent

3. What type of matrix is used in the placement of a Class III composite restoration?

    a. universal matrix band

    b. plastic matrix strip

    c. crown matrix form

    d. sectional matrix

4. What can the matrix strip be made of when used with a composite or glass ionomer?

    a. nylon

    b. acetate

    c. celluloid

    d. all of these

5. What does the etchant remove from the surface of the dentin to improve the bonding?

   a. smear layer
   b. enamel
   c. biofilm
   d. cementum

6. Which type of composite has a filler size from 1 to 3 microns, is fracture resistant, and is a good choice for a Class IV restoration?

   a. macrofill
   b. microfill
   c. hybrid
   d. nanofill

7. Which is the sequence of use of materials for placing Class III composite restoration?

   a. bonding agent, mylar matrix strip, selection of shade, abrasive strips
   b. abrasive strips, bonding agent, mylar matrix strip, shade
   c. shade, bonding agent, abrasive strips, mylar matrix strip
   d. shade guide, mylar matrix strip, bonding agent, abrasive strips

8. How should etchant, bonding agent and composite resin be stored?

   a. in a dedicated refrigerator
   b. at room temperature
   c. temperature close to body temperature
   d. by manufacturer's directions

9. A patient has an incisal chip on tooth 8. Which composite is a good choice because it is a cosmetic filling material, 0.01 to 0.1 microns, and resistant to abrasion?

   a. macrofill
   b. microfill
   c. hybrid
   d. nanofill

10. Which are used to shape and finish a Class III composite restoration?

   a. diamonds
   b. finishing burs
   c. abrasive strips
   d. all of these

CHAPTER APPLICATION

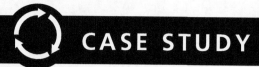
CASE STUDY

Amber is scheduled for a composite restoration in today's appointment. There are many types of materials the dentist has to choose from. Amber needs a distal filling on tooth 8 and a disto-occlusal on tooth 30.

1. What type(s) of composites would be placed for a restoration on tooth 8 as compared to the restoration placed on tooth 30?

_____

_____

_____

2. What are the properties that make a composite material ideal for Amber's restorations?

_____

_____

_____

X Critical Thinking

The treatment of the cavity preparation prior to the placement of the composite restoration varies based on the amount of enamel and dentin removed and how close the prep is to the pulp.

1. What materials should be placed before the composite restoration if the dentin has been exposed?

_____

_____

2. If there is a near pulp exposure, what materials should be placed before the composite restoration?

_____

_____

3. Name the esthetic restorative material that has a similar placement technique to composite, and describe the differences.

_____

_____

_____

CHAPTER 33

Dental Laboratory Material

SPECIFIC INSTRUCTIONAL OBJECTIVES

At the completion of this chapter, you will be able to meet these objectives:

1. Use terms presented in this chapter.

2. Distinguish between alginates and alginate substitutes.

3. Describe factors that can influence working and setting times for alginates.

4. Demonstrate the knowledge and skills needed to prepare, take, and remove alginate impressions and wax bites.

5. Explain why an alginate impression must be stored properly.

6. Describe the uses of elastomeric impression materials.

7. Distinguish between polyvinyl siloxane and polyether impression materials.

8. Demonstrate the knowledge and skills necessary to prepare elastomeric impression materials such as polysulfide, silicone (polysiloxane and polyvinyl siloxanes), and polyether for the dentist.

9. Compare and contrast different types of gypsum materials.

10. Discuss the materials necessary for fabrication of diagnostic casts.

11. Explain how excess water affects the manipulation and properties of gypsum materials.

12. Demonstrate the knowledge and skills necessary to pour and trim a diagnostic cast.

13. Identify use of a dental articulator and facebow for dental casts or study models.

14. Demonstrate taking a facebow transfer and mounting models on an articulator.

15. Identify various classifications and uses of waxes used in dentistry.

16. Identify the differences and similarities in techniques of the common methods of fabricating custom-made impression trays.

17. Demonstrate the knowledge and skills necessary to fabricate and fit custom temporary restorations.

18. Identify the two types of provisional materials.

19. Identify properties of provisional materials and indicate their clinical importance.

VOCABULARY BUILDER

Matching

Match each term with the appropriate definition.

1. _____ dimensional change

2. _____ catalyst

3. _____ beading

4. _____ invert

5. _____ imbibition

6. _____ monomer

7. _____ thermoplastic

8. _____ spatulation

9. _____ polymerization

10. _____ gelatin time

a. method by which elastomeric impression material sets

b. a compound whose molecules can join together to form a polymer

c. paste portion of elastomeric impression material that reacts with the base paste

d. the amount of time it takes for the material to solidify

e. action used to mix alginate impression material by hand

f. an elevation that is made of wax around the border of a tissue surface of a tray

g. measurement used to determine accuracy of impression material

h. ability of alginate impression to absorb water if stored in water

i. pour method refers to pouring both the anatomic and the art portions of the model in one step

CHAPTER REVIEW

Multiple Choice

1. Alginate impressions make which type of mold?

   a. negative
   b. positive
   c. sol
   d. agar-agar

2. Alginate is considered which type of impression material?

   a. reversible hydrocolloid
   b. irreversible hydrocolloid
   c. polysulfide
   d. gypsum

3. If an impression loses water content due to heat, dryness, or exposure to air, shrinkage occurs, a condition known as

   a. imbibition.
   b. exothermic reaction.
   c. polymerization.
   d. syneresis.

4. What is the process by which the catalyst and accelerator begin to cure?

   a. exothermic reaction
   b. polymerization
   c. distortion
   d. calcination

5. Which of the following is not an elastomeric impression material?

   a. silicone

   b. agar-agar

   c. polyether

   d. polysulfide

6. Which type of gypsum is for model or laboratory plaster?

   a. Type I

   b. Type II

   c. Type III

   d. Type IV

7. Which material is an elastomeric impression material that is available in putty form and is used for making a custom tray?

   a. silicone

   b. polyether

   c. polysulfide

   d. methacrylate

8. Which is the ingredient that accelerates or starts the process of setting the impression material?

   a. catalyst

   b. base

   c. monomer

   d. polymer

9. What equipment is used to duplicate the function of the temporomandibular joint?

   a. facebow and articulator

   b. study model and bite rims

   c. custom tray and articulator

   d. study model and custom tray

10. Utility wax is used to bead around trays to extend them. Under which of the following groups of waxes would utility wax be classified?

   a. impression

   b. processing

   c. pattern

   d. custom

True or False

Circle whether the answer is true or false.

1. Plaster particles are more irregular and require more water to wet each surface of each particle. The ratio of water to powder for plaster is 30 mL of water to 100g of powder.

   a. Both statements are true.

   b. Both statements are false.

   c. The first statement is true; the second statement is false.

   a. The first statement is false; the second statement is true.

2. For the double-pour, the anatomical portion of the cast is mixed and poured first, after which a second mix is made and the base (art) portion is poured.

   a. Both statements are true.

   b. Both statements are false.

   c. The first statement is true; the second statement is false.

   d. The first statement is false; the second statement is true.

3. Preformed aluminum temporary crowns are used on the posterior teeth because they lack esthetic value. They are only made without any anatomy and resemble thimbles with parallel straight sides and flat, occlusal surfaces.

   a. Both statements are true.

   b. Both statements are false.

   c. The first statement is true; the second statement is false.

   d. The first statement is false; the second statement is true.

4. **T   F**   When trimming a cast, draw a rounded line from canine to canine and make the cut for the maxillary cast.

25. **T   F**   Due to the taste, staining, and long setting time, polyether materials are not used as often anymore and have been replaced with polysulfide materials.

26. **T   F**   For a polysulfide impression, the mixing and loading time must be completed in 4 minutes.

Matching

Match the gypsum material to the water-to-powder ratio.

1. _____ Type I: Impression Plaster

2. _____ Type II: Laboratory or model plaster

3. _____ Type III: Laboratory stone

4. _____ Type IV: Die stone

   a. 100 g powder/30 mL water

   b. 100 g powder/60 mL water

   c. 100 g powder/24 mL water

   d. 100 g powder/50 mL water

CERTIFICATION REVIEW

Multiple Choice

1. Gypsum materials include which of the following?

   1. plaster

   2. Type I stone

   3. polysulfide

   4. silicone

      a. 1, 2, 3

      b. 1, 2

      c. 1 only

      d. 3, 4

2. Which of the following is used to avoid seating a custom tray too deeply?

   a. stops

   b. resin

   c. liner

   d. wax

3. Alginate is used mostly for which type of impression?

   a. custom

   b. provisional

   c. preliminary

   d. irreversible

4. Plaster is a form of which material?

   a. gypsum
   b. hydrocolloid
   c. elastomeric
   d. provisional

5. Which of the following are advantages of using reversible hydrocolloid?

   1. more accurate than alginate
   2. comparatively economical after initial equipment purchase
   3. can be used for impressions for crown and bridge construction
   4. less equipment needed
   5. less setting time required
   6. not affected by atmospheric conditions
      a. 1, 4, 5
      b. 1, 2, 6
      c. 1, 2, 3
      d. 2, 3, 4

6. Which of the following equipment and supplies would indicate the taking of a polysulfide impression?

   1. custom tray painted with adhesive
   2. water measure
   3. glass slab
   4. two pastes, base and catalyst
   5. rubber bowl
   6. mixing tip
      a. 2, 3, 5
      b. 2, 3, 6
      c. 1, 4, 6
      d. 1, 2, 3

7. The amount of water used when mixing type III dental stone should be

   a. 50.
   b. 30.
   c. 60.
   d. 23.

8. The depth of the base (art) portion of a trimmed diagnostic model should be which of the following in comparison to the entire depth of the model?

   a. 1/3
   b. 1/2
   c. 2/3
   d. 1/4

9. Which of the following is an ideal feature of an alginate impression material?

   a. sets in 30 seconds
   b. flexible, easy to remove from the mouth
   c. good accuracy
   d. sharp detail

10. When choosing an impression tray, which of the following should be considered?

    a. choose a tray that fits snuggly around teeth

    b. choose a tray that leaves about 4 mm of space between teeth and tray
    c. choose a tray that is metal rather than plastic
    d. choose a tray that covers the most distal tooth or tuberosities

CHAPTER APPLICATION

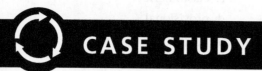

CASE STUDY

Felix is a patient having a first molar prepared for a crown; the molar which is the largest tooth in the mouth, and Felix's molar is no exception. The dentist has directed the dental assistant to fabricate and place the provisional restoration for Felix using the direct matrix technique.

1. Which is true of the direct matrix technique?

_____

2. Which would be the first step?

_____

Critical Thinking

1. Optimal storage of alginate is in a cool, dry place. If it is kept in an area where moisture can contaminate it, what is likely to happen?

_____

2. The most commonly used trays are the perforated trays that come in metal and plastic. Why are these trays perforated?

_____

3. Why do we take a bite-wax registration?

_____

_____

4. What is the use for a facebow and articulator?

_____

5. What are the two types of provisional restorations?

_____

6. What is the difference between a direct and indirect matrix technique?

_____

_____

7. Where does the operator stand when taking a maxillary and mandibular alginate impression?

_____

8. There is a unique difference between reversible and irreversible hydrocolloid material regarding the setting reaction. What is this difference?

_____

_____

Assist with Comprehensive Patient Care

CHAPTER 34

Pediatrics

SPECIFIC INSTRUCTIONAL OBJECTIVES

At the completion of this chapter, you will be able to meet these objectives:

1. Use terms presented in this chapter.
2. Discuss need for pediatrics as a specialty and the pediatric environment.
3. Describe differences in pediatric dental caries.
4. Summarize what occurs during a pediatric oral exam.
5. Outline a good pediatric preventive program.
6. Explain special behavior management techniques for various stages of child development and patients with special needs.
7. Summarize special procedures performed in a pediatric practice.
8. Compare and contrast pulpotomy and pulpectomy procedures.
9. Defend the need for pediatric orthodontic treatment.
10. Describe common traumatic injuries and related treatment.

VOCABULARY BUILDER

Matching

Match each term with the appropriate definition.

1. _____ –tomy   a. dislocate

2. _____ –ectomy   b. tooth erupts in abnormal position

3. _____ ankylose   c. partial surgical removal

4. _____ avulse   d. to thrust outward

5. _____ concuss   e. complete surgical removal

6. _____ extrude	f. to push with force
7. _____ luxate	g. injury due to violent blow
8. _____ thrust	h. to grow together
9. _____ congenital	i. born with
10. _____ ectopic	j. forcible tearing away

11. _____ mandate	a. desired behavior
12. _____ pulpectomy	b. number of years old
13. _____ rampant	c. widespread
14. _____ sequelae	d. partial removal of pulp
15. _____ bifida	e. to require
16. _____ pulpotomy	f. measure of development in mind
17. _____ chronological age	g. anything that follows something else
18. _____ emotional age	h. measure of maturity of feelings
19. _____ maturity age	i. split spine
20. _____ modeling	j. remove all of the pulp

CHAPTER REVIEW

True or False

Circle whether the answer is true or false.

1. **T   F**   The AAPD recommend that an infant be weaned from the breast or bottle by the time they are 6 months old.

2. **T   F**   General anesthesia is administered to a child in a hospital or outpatient hospital setting.

3. **T   F**   A crossbite is recorded when the maxillary teeth are facial to the mandibular teeth.

4. **T   F**   Primary teeth should be reimplanted as soon as possible after an avulsion.

5. **T   F**   The first step is stopping bleeding after an orofacial soft tissue trauma is direct pressure against the site for 10 minutes.

6. If a small child eats an excessive amount of toothpaste from the tube, milk or yogurt can be given the child to reduce the immediate symptoms. The toothpaste needs to be stored out of the child's reach to prevent potential enamel fluorosis.

   a. Both statements are true.
   b. Both statements are false.
   c. The first statement is true; the second statement is false.
   d. The first statement is false; the second statement is true.

7. **T**   **F**   Amalgam, composite resin, and glass ionomer restorations can only be used on permanent teeth.

8. **T**   **F**   Most pediatric dentists use veneered steel crowns when full coverage for an anterior teeth is needed.

9. **T**   **F**   The medication formocresol is placed after the pulpotomy to cauterize the remaining pulp tissue.

10. **T**   **F**   Primate spacing of erupted primary teeth allows adequate space for erupting permanent teeth.

Multiple Choice

1. Which is a unique characteristic of primary teeth versus permanent?

    a. thinner enamel
    b. shallower pulp chamber

    c. exfoliation
    d. all of these

2. What space maintainer is used when the primary second molar is missing and the permanent molar as not erupted?

    a. band and loop
    b. lingual arch

    c. distal shoe
    d. retainer

3. A behavior management technique called _____ consists of telling the child the name of the instrument, showing it to the child, and then demonstrating how it is used.

    a. voice control
    b. tell, show, and do

    c. subjective
    d. nonverbal

4. The _____ behavior management technique pairs a timid child in the dental chair with a cooperative child of similar age.

    a. positive reinforcement
    b. distraction

    c. modeling
    d. nonverbal communication

5. Children who are involved in contact sports should be fitted for

    a. fixed space maintainers.
    b. removable space maintainers.

    c. dental matrices.
    d. mouth guards.

6. Behavior modification is sometimes necessary. Fixed appliances, such as cribs and rakes, are used to prevent

    a. thumb sucking.
    b. tongue thrust.

    c. modeling.
    d. pulpotomy.

7. Which custom matrix is designed for and used on primary teeth?

    a. T-band
    b. Tofflemire

    c. space maintainer
    d. stainless steel crown

8. Which procedure is performed on young permanent teeth to leave part of the pulp intact, maintain pulp vitality, and allow enough time for the root end to develop and close?

    a. direct pulp capping
    b. pulpectomy

    c. pulpotomy
    d. root canal therapy

9. For which of the following reasons is the primary dentition restored?

    a. Primary teeth are needed to hold space for the permanent teeth.
    b. Primary teeth maintain the functions of the teeth in chewing, speech, and aesthetics.

c. Primary teeth act as guides for the permanent dentition during eruption.

d. all of the above

10. The following general behavior characteristics fit children of which age?

1. can respond to the dentist's instructions
2. can understand simple explanations
3. like to be with parents and siblings
4. like to play, for example, "see the 'squirt gun'"
   a. 4 to 6
   c. 2 to 4
   b. 2 to 6
   d. 6 to 12

CERTIFICATION REVIEW

Multiple Choice

1. When may patient be referred to a pediatric dentist?

a. an anxious or uncooperative child

b. a child with special needs

c. a child with rampant caries or oral developmental problems

d. all of these

2. What is the number one childhood disease according to the U.S. Surgeon General's Report?

a. measles

b. meningitis

c. dental caries

d. obesity

3. At what age is it recommended that a child first sees a dentist?

a. 6 months

b. 12 months

c. 18 months

d. 24 months

4. How should the dental assistant communicate with a child patient?

a. Talk to them as they would an adult.

b. Be strict and explain the office rules.

c. It is best to talk to the child through the parent.

d. Be friendly but firm.

5. How is child abuse or neglect handled in the dental office by the dentist and dental assistant?

a. Document suspicious signs for future reference only.

b. Have a discussion with the parent.

c. It is not something handled in the dental office.

d. They are legally mandated to report suspected child abuse or neglect.

6. Which term is used by the Academy of Pediatric Dentistry to describes the presence of rapid cavitation in a child 71 month or younger?

   a. nursing bottle syndrome

   b. rampant caries

   c. early childhood caries

   d. baby bottle tooth decay

7. Which teeth are usually the first teeth to be exfoliated?

   a. A and J

   b. K and T

   c. E and F

   d. O and P

8. What primary teeth do teeth 3 and 14 replace?

   a. A and J

   b. B and I

   c. K and T

   d. erupt behind A and J

9. After adjusting the height of an SSC, what instrument is used to smooth the edges?

   a. crown and bridge scissors

   b. 112 pliers

   c. green stone

   d. prophy brush

10. A primary tooth is severely decayed, and the nerve is involved. What procedure would be performed to remove just the coronal portion of the pulp?

   a. root canal therapy

   b. partial root canal therapy

   c. pulpectomy

   d. pulpotomy

CHAPTER APPLICATION

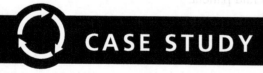

CASE STUDY

Joel, age 4, has kept his parents up at night with toothaches. His parents took him to their general dentist, and it was not a pleasant experience! Joel would not open his mouth and would scream when the dentist approached his mouth. The general dentist referred him to a pediatric dentist.

1. List some general behavior characteristics of children at age 4.

   _____

   _____

   _____

2. Name and describe some nonpharmacological behavior management techniques.

_____

_____

_____

_____

_____

_____

_____

_____

_____

_____

_____

3. If the dentist decides that pharmacological behavior management will be needed to treat an uncooperative patient, what are some medications that are used to sedate a child during the dental treatment?

_____

_____

_____

✗ Critical Thinking

Accepting a role as a pediatric assistant means different duties and responsibilities than in a general practice. Describe the dental assistant's role and responsibilities in a pediatric dental office.

1. Describe the characteristics of a successful pediatric dental assistant.

_____

_____

2. Describe the dental assistant's role and responsibilities in a pediatric dental office.

_____

_____

_____

_____

CHAPTER 35

Orthodontics

SPECIFIC INSTRUCTIONAL OBJECTIVES

At the completion of this chapter, you will be able to meet these objectives:

1. Use terms presented in this chapter.
2. Describe the role and responsibilities of each member of the orthodontic team.
3. Discuss the purpose of each section of an orthodontic new patient exam.
4. Explain the four planes of space when evaluating the occlusion and skeletal patterns.
5. Describe three etiological factors in the cause of a malocclusion.
6. Summarize the process of developing a diagnosis and an orthodontic treatment plan by the orthodontist.
7. List each orthodontic diagnostic record that is needed for diagnosis and orthodontic treatment planning.
8. Describe the steps in conducting a treatment plan consultation with a patient.
9. Describe the types of orthodontic treatment provided to young children.
10. Describe the types of orthodontic treatment of adolescents including the use of growth appliances.
11. Describe the types of orthodontic treatment of adults including clear aligner therapy and orthognathic surgery.
12. Discuss the purpose and types of orthodontic retention of the final result.
13. Sequence comprehensive orthodontic treatment appointments.

VOCABULARY BUILDER

Matching

Match each term with the appropriate definition.

1. _____ pro
2. _____ retro
3. _____ gnath
4. _____ cleft
5. _____ brux
6. _____ fraction
7. _____ incline

a. opening
b. into sections
c. backward
d. lean
e. jaw
f. gnash teeth
g. forward

8. _____ proclination
9. _____ retroclination
10. _____ separators
11. _____ transverse
12. _____ perimeter
13. _____ retainer
14. _____ underbite
15. _____ overjet

a. maxillary incisors overlap the mandibular incisors
b. extending from side to side
c. forward leaning relation
d. keeps tooth in proper position
e. backward leaning relation
f. spacers
g. measure around
h. mandibular incisors overlap maxillary incisors

Fill in the Blank

Please fill in the blank with one of the choices provided.

bracket   abrafactions   retrognathism

deleterious   asymmetry

1. The assistant noted the _____ that caused the loss of tooth structure due to forces from chewing.

2. When the right and left sides of the face are not equal, it is called _____.

3. The _____ keeps the arch wire in place.

4. When one or both of the jaws are posterior to their normal positions, it is called _____.

5. A situation is _____ when it is harmful or injurious to the patient's health.

CHAPTER REVIEW

True or False

Circle whether the answer is true or false.

1. **T   F**   Maxillary and mandibular teeth are in maximum contact and normally spaced in an ideal occlusion relationship.

2. **T   F**   The ligature wire wraps around the bracket and is tightened by twisting.

3. **T   F**   The bionator is used to position the lower jaw forward and to encourage lower jaw growth.

4. **T   F**   Zinc phosphate cement is preferred over a glass ionomer cement due to its ionic bonding.

5. **T   F**   Clear aligners can correct a skeletal problem in a growing patient.

Matching

Match the orthodontic instrument with its function.

1. _____ Howe pliers   a. adjusts and bends wire and clasps

2. _____ bird-beak pliers   b. removes excess cement

3. _____ three-prong pliers   c. utility plier

4. _____ tweed loop pliers   d. places the arch wire

5. _____ scaler   e. contours wire and forms springs

6. _____ needle holder (Mathieu)   f. forms loops and springs in wire

7. _____ Weingart utility pliers   g. guides arch wire into place and places elastics

Multiple Choice

1. The orthodontic team consists of the

   1. scheduling coordinator.
   2. records coordinator.
   3. chairside assistant.
   4. financial coordinator.

      a. 1, 2, 3   c. 1, 3, 4
      b. 2, 3, 4   d. 1, 2, 3, 4

2. Who established the system for classifying malocclusion?

   a. Black   c. Pasteur
   b. Angle   d. Bolton

3. Which is (are) an example of a fixed orthodontic appliance?

   a. a retainer   c. braces
   b. an activator   d. headgear

4. Which fixed appliance is either welded to the bands or bonded directly to the teeth?

   a. band   c. buccal tube
   b. bracket   d. ligature wire

5. The function of (the) _____ is to apply force to move the teeth into or to hold the teeth in the desired positions.

   a. buccal tubes
   b. bracket
   c. arch wire
   d. springs

6. Which removable appliance, usually worn for a specific number of hours each day, is used to apply force to move teeth, and to restrain or alter cranial-facial bone growth?

   a. space maintainer
   b. headgear
   c. activator
   d. tooth positioner

7. Which are placed in the contact areas between the teeth, forcing the teeth to spread to accommodate the orthodontic bands?

   a. separators
   b. plastic rings
   c. brackets
   d. springs

8. What is the vertical overlap of the maxillary and mandibular anterior teeth?

   a. overjet
   b. overbite
   c. underjet
   d. crossbite

9. The horizontal distance between the labial surface of the mandibular anterior teeth and the lingual surface of the maxillary anterior teeth is called a(an)

   a. overjet.
   b. overbite.
   c. open bite.
   d. crossbite.

10. Which type of imaging has allowed orthodontists to provide treatment without the need to create study models?

    a. digital intraoral scan
    b. three-dimensional
    c. panoramic
    d. cephalometric

11. Who invented the self-ligating bracket?

    a. Damon
    b. Angle
    c. Frankel
    d. Herbst

12. Which type of wire is most often used toward the end of treatment as a finishing wire, when more control of tooth movement is needed?

    a. beta-titanium
    b. nickel-titanium
    c. gold
    d. stainless steel

13. The etiology of malocclusion can fall into one of three categories: genetic, systemic, or local. For which of the following might genetic factors be responsible?

    1. systemic diseases
    2. trauma
    3. palatal clefts
    4. supernumerary teeth
    5. thumb sucking
    6. nutritional disturbances

    a. 1, 2
    b. 3, 4
    c. 5, 6
    d. 3, 6

14. Ideal occlusion includes the following:

 1. Maxillary first molar mesiobuccal cusp fits between the mandibular first molar and second premolar.
 2. Maxillary first molar mesiobuccal cusp fits into the buccal groove of the mandibular first molar.
 3. Teeth may be slightly rotated and turned.
 4. Anterior teeth overlap by 2 mm maxillary to mandibular.

    a. 1, 4   c. 2, 4

    b. 1, 3   d. 2, 3, 4

CERTIFICATION REVIEW

Multiple Choice

1. What type of orthodontic treatment involves using a fixed or removable appliance for a crossbite?

 a. preventive
 b. interceptive
 c. corrective
 d. comprehensive

2. Which classification shows the mesiobuccal cusp of the maxillary first molar meeting mesial to the mesiobuccal groove of the mandibular first molar?

 a. neutrocclusion
 b. Class I
 c. Class II
 d. Class III

3. What is the tooth relationship when the maxillary incisors stick out in front of the mandibular incisors?

 a. open bite
 b. overjet
 c. underbite
 d. crossbite

4. When using the Angle Classification to identify a patient's occlusal relationship, which teeth relationships are used?

 a. second molars and second premolars
 b. first molars and central incisors
 c. second molars and canines
 d. first molars and canines

5. Which classification has proclined maxillary anterior incisors?

 a. Class I
 b. Class II
 c. Class III
 d. Class I and III

6. What is the ideal overbite?

    a. 1 mm
    b. 2 mm
    c. 3 mm
    d. 4 mm

7. Which may be the cause of malocclusion?

    a. genetics
    b. systemic disease
    c. oral habits
    d. all of these

8. A protraction headgear may be used to correct which classification?

    a. Class I
    b. Class II
    c. Class III
    d. Class I and II

9. What is tied around the brackets to hold arch wires in place?

    a. elastics
    b. ligature wires
    c. separators
    d. rubber bands

10. Which describes when the maxillary and mandibular jaws are in a closed position that produces maximum contact?

    a. centric occlusion
    b. neutral occlusion
    c. malocclusion
    d. Class I occlusion

CHAPTER APPLICATION

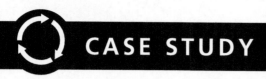

CASE STUDY

As a child, Lynwood struggled with an underbite; he experienced difficulty in chewing food, and kids teasing him. Now an adult, he is concerned about his facial profile for the work that he does, which has motivated him to seek help. The general dentist has referred Lynwood to an orthodontist.

1. Describe an underbite.

   _____

   _____

   _____

2. Name and describe the facial profile of a patient with an underbite.

   _____

   _____

   _____

3. What classification does Lynwood have?

   _____

   _____

   _____

4. What treatment may be needed?

   _____

   _____

   _____

X Critical Thinking

1. Being efficient means that the assistant is ready to perform specific tasks in the orthodontic treatment sequence. Sequence the steps in the direct bonding brackets procedure.

   _____

   _____

CHAPTER **36**

Oral and Maxillofacial Surgery

VOCABULARY BUILDER

Matching I

Match each term with the appropriate definition.

1. _____ arthroscopy

2. _____ subluxate

3. _____ luxate

4. _____ arthroplasty

5. _____ anxiolysis

a. to dislocate or displace a joint

b. any class of drugs that reduces anxiety

c. scope used to diagnose an injury or disease of a joint

d. to partially dislocate

e. surgical repair of a joint

Fill in the Blank

Please fill in the blank with one of the choices provided.

(grafting, wet socket, TMD, parasthesia, dry socket, gingivoplasty)

1. Alveolitis is an inflammation or an infection of the socket, also known as _____.

2. Transplanting tissue from one site on the body is known as _____.

3. Tinnitus is a ringing or buzzing in the ear, which could be a symptom of _____.

Matching II

1. _____ -plasty   a. surgical shaping

2. _____ arthro-   b. inflammation

3. _____ -tis   c. joint

4. _____ gnath   d. jaw

CHAPTER REVIEW

True or False

Circle whether the answer is true or false.

1. **T   F**   Oral and maxillofacial surgery is one of the nine recognized dental specialties by the American Dental Association.

2. **T   F**   Universal forceps can be used on any of the four quadrants.

3. **T   F**   During procedures performed in a sterile environment, one surgical assistant is on duty.

4. **T   F**   Treatment of diabetic patients should be performed in the evening.

5. **T   F**   Unless excessive bleeding occurs, sutures are rarely used.

6. **T   F**   Postoperative swelling is managed by the application of heat as directed.

Multiple Choice

1. Procedures often performed in a hospital operating room setting include the following *except*

   a. TMJ surgery.   c. extraction.
   b. cleft palate surgery.   d. jaw reconstruction.

2. A drug-induced state during which a patient remains conscious and is able to maintain a patent airway is which type of sedation?

   a. minimal   c. deep
   b. moderate   d. anxiolysis

3. Oral and maxillofacial surgery involves surgery for

   a. functional malformations.   c. facial aesthetics.
   b. facial injuries.   d. all of the above

4. The surgical dental assistant would perform all the following tasks *except*

   a. transfer instruments.

   b. administer local anesthetic.

   c. maintain the operating field during procedures.

   d. take vital signs.

5. The most common site for development of a dry socket is

   a. first molars.

   b. maxillary cuspids.

   c. third molars.

   d. mandibular cuspids.

6. Patients who are more prone to developing alveolitis include all of the following, *except*

   a. smokers.

   b. patients with excessive trauma during surgery.

   c. patients taking birth control pills.

   d. patients taking osteoporosis medications.

7. Procedures often performed in a hospital operating room setting include the following *except*

   a. TMJ surgery.

   b. cleft palate surgery.

   c. extraction.

   d. jaw reconstruction.

8. When a blade removal device is not available, which of the following can be used to insert and remove the blade from the handle?

   a. hemostat

   b. needle holder

   c. college pliers

   d. rongeurs

9. This a contouring process in which sharp edges and points on the alveolar ridge are contoured and smoothed.

   a. alveolitis

   b. osseointegration

   c. exodontia

   d. alveoplasty

10. A nonsurgical procedure that involves the oral surgeon removing a layer of cells from the surface lesion is called a(an)

   a. incisional biopsy.

   b. excisional biopsy.

   c. dental implant.

   d. exfoliative cytology.

11. The most common complication following an extraction is

   a. luxation.

   b. alveoplasty.

   c. alveolitis.

   d. exfoliative cytology.

12. Extracted teeth are disposed of in the

   a. regular waste.

   b. sharps container.

   c. biohazard container.

   d. none of the above

13. One of the most common procedures the oral surgeon performs is a(n)

   a. composite restoration.

   b. amalgam restoration.

   c. fixed prosthetic.

   d. third molar extraction.

14. The receptionist and the business staff play an important part in the oral surgery office. Which of the following are duties of the office staff?

   a. communications from the referring dentist

   b. financial arrangements

   c. insurance claims

   d. all of the above

15. Surgery to relieve pain and restore range of motion by realigning or reconstructing a joint is called

    a. arthroplasty.
    b. articular eminence recontouring.

    c. arthrocentesis.
    d. arthroscopy.

16. Which type of imaging technology can aid the surgeon in treating patients with severe trauma?

    a. panoramic imaging
    b. cephalometric imaging

    c. magnetic resonance imaging
    d. 3D cone beam imaging

17. Which of the following procedures might an expanded functions dental assistant perform?

    a. remove sutures
    b. perform a biopsy

    c. take and record vital signs
    d. stabilize the patient's head and mandible during surgery

18. Which of the following instruments hold the lip, tongue, and cheeks so the operator can view site during a procedure?

    a. periosteal elevator
    b. retractor

    c. straight elevator
    d. surgical curette

CERTIFICATION REVIEW

Multiple Choice

1. When performing suture removal, which of the following should be prevented?

    a. pulling the knot through the tissue
    b. using antiseptic on the tissue

    c. cutting below the suture knot
    d. retaining resorbable suture

2. In what sort of biopsy does the oral surgeon remove a small section of a lesion and include a small border of normal tissue?

    a. excisional
    b. incisional

    c. exfoliative
    d. extraction

3. To control swelling in the first 24 hours after a surgical procedure, the patient should be advised to

    a. apply ice packs, alternating 20 minutes on and 20 minutes off.
    b. bite on gauze with firm pressure for 30 minutes.
    c. rinse with warm salt water.
    d. apply moist heat every 20 minutes.

4. To prevent alveolitis after a tooth extraction, the patient should be instructed to

    a. apply ice packs.
    b. rinse as often as possible.

    c. take anti-inflammatories.
    d. avoid drinking through a straw.

5. The tray setup for the treatment of alveolitis would include

    a. a local anesthetic syringe.
    b. iodoform gauze.

    c. a surgical aspirating tip.
    d. a bite block.

6. Which of the following would be included in the setup for the removal of an impacted third molar?

    a. finishing burs
    b. high volume evacuation tip

    c. greater number of blades
    d. high speed handpiece

7. Which of the following would be included in the setup for the removal of sutures

   a. rongeurs

   b. hemostat

   c. surgical aspirating tip

   d. sterile saline water

8. Which of the following would be included in the setup for a routine extraction?

   a. finishing burs

   b. high volume evacuation tip

   c. scalpel and blade

   d. surgical curette

9. Which of the following instruments hold the lip, tongue, and cheeks so the operator can view the site during a procedure?

   a. periosteal elevator

   b. retractor

   c. straight elevator

   d. surgical curette

10. Which of the following instruments loosens the tooth for removal?

   a. periosteal elevator

   b. retractor

   c. straight elevator

   d. surgical curette

CHAPTER APPLICATION

CASE STUDY 1

Donald has had an alveoplasty, and the anesthesia is wearing off. He is glad that the dental team sent him home with postoperative instructions and a written appointment date. He was so groggy that he does not remember much of what they had told him at the office.

1. Describe how postoperative home care instructions are provided.

   _____

2. List what to do following an extraction.

   _____

   _____

3. List five activities and substances that are to be avoided following an extraction.

   _____

   _____

   _____

   _____

   _____

4. If a patient still has questions, who should they contact?

   _____

5. How long do resorbable sutures take until they resorb?

   _____

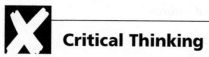

Critical Thinking

1. Following the administration of local anesthesia, what is the first step in the procedure for a routine extraction?

_____

_____

_____

_____

2. When are extracted teeth not subject to provisions of the OSHA Bloodborne Pathogens Standards?

_____

_____

3. State the differences between an incisional and excisional biopsy procedure.

_____

_____

_____

_____

4. Why is it important for a malformation such as a cleft palate be repaired?

_____

_____

5. List the common signs for TMD.

_____

_____

_____

CHAPTER 37

Endodontics

SPECIFIC INSTRUCTIONAL OBJECTIVES

At the completion of this chapter, you will be able to meet these objectives:

1. Use terms presented in this chapter.
2. Recognize the anatomy of the pulpal tissues.
3. Describe the progression of pulpal disease.
4. Discuss periradicular and pulpal involvement conditions.
5. Describe diagnostic procedures relating to the treatment of pulpal disease.
6. Explain the difference between a tooth needing a nonsurgical endodontic procedure versus a surgical endodontic procedure.
7. Summarize the steps in completing root canal therapy.
8. Describe the appearance of intracanal instruments.
9. Explain the use of intracanal instruments.
10. Indicate the necessary postoperative instructions that should be given to the patient immediately following the root canal therapy appointment.
11. Discuss surgical endodontic procedures.

VOCABULARY BUILDER

Matching

Match each term with the appropriate definition.

1. _____ acute pulpitis

2. _____ apexogenisis

3. _____ extirpate

a. irreversible inflammation of the pulp

b. a form of localized nodular of inflammatory cells found in tissues

c. procedure with reversible pulpitis leaving pulp in root to stimulate the process of development of the apex

4. _____ chronic pulpitis   d. sudden and severe inflammation of the pulp

5. _____ granuloma   e. to remove by surgery

Fill in the Blank

Please fill in the blank with one of the choices provided.

(Endodontia, pulpal, residual, parulis, cyst, grafting, periapical, residual, neoplasm)

1. If a granuloma is left untreated and the irritation continues, a ____ forms.

2. A small abscess on the gum that originates in an abscess in the pulp of a tooth is known as a _____.

3. A small radiolucency (typically less than 1 cm) is a _____ cyst. If the cyst remains after the tooth is extracted, it is considered _____.

4. _____ is a term pertaining to the inner part of the tooth.

5. Surgical removal of a _____ would be inevitable as it would grow and cause more alveolar bone destruction.

CHAPTER REVIEW

Multiple Choice

1. Which of the following procedures is dealt with and included in the branch of dentistry called endodontics?

   a. diagnosis   c. periapical surgery
   b. root canal treatment   d. all of the above

2. The endodontic bender is designed to bend all of the following *except*

   a. reamers.   c. burs.
   b. files.   d. pluggers.

3. Which instrument is used to remove excess gutta percha?

   a. spreader   c. plugger
   b. Glick 1   d. spoon

4. Which of the following instruments has a long, twisted shank and blades that are far apart, and is used in a twisting motion?

   a. file   c. reamer
   b. broach   d. Gates–Glidden drill

5. A thermoplastic material that is flexible at room temperature and is used to fill the canal is which of the following?

   a. rubber stop   c. gutta percha
   b. file stop   d. marker

6. Which of these is a material that comes in powder or liquid form, is thick when mixed, is used with obturating materials, and is inserted in the canal?

    a. gutta percha
    b. sealer

    c. paper points
    d. marker

7. Which piece of equipment measures the distance to the apex of the tooth and displays the information on a digital readout?

    a. vitality scanner
    b. pulp tester

    c. heating unit
    d. apex finder

8. During which phase of endodontic treatment is the pulp canal restored by being filled and sealed permanently?

    a. reversible pulpitis
    b. pulpotomy

    c. obturation
    d. hemisection

9. The master cone material is which of the following?

    a. paper point
    b. Lentulo spiral

    c. calcium hydroxide
    d. gutta percha

10. In which procedure are the apex of the root and the infection surrounding the area surgically removed?

    a. amputation
    b. hemisection

    c. pulpectomy
    d. apicoectomy

11. Which of the following are characteristics of intracanal instruments?

    1. precise diameters
    2. precise lengths
    3. made of stainless steel
    4. made of nickel titanium alloy wire
    5. gutta percha
    6. flexible
    7. fracture resistant
    8. corrosion resistant

    a. 1, 2, 3, 4, 5, 6, 7, 8
    b. 1, 2, 3, 5, 8

    c. 1, 2, 3, 4, 6, 7, 8
    d. 1, 2, 5, 6, 7, 8

True or False

Circle whether the answer is true or false.

1. When using an electronic pulp tester, If the patient first feels the current in the control tooth at setting 5 but feels current below setting 5 on the tooth in question, that tooth is hypersensitive. If the control tooth feels current at 5 and the tooth being tested only feels current above 5, the tooth is losing sensitivity and is possibly necrotic.

    a. Both statements are true.
    b. Both statements are false.
    c. The first statement is true; the second statement is false.
    d. The first statement is false; the second statement is true.

2. **T   F**   During a pulpotomy, all the pulp is removed from within the coronal pulp chamber.

3. **T   F**   When there is an infection in the pulp tissue, the only treatment option is root canal therapy.

4. Hand intracanal instruments (reamers and files), power-assisted instruments, and intracanal solutions are used in debridement of the pulp canals. Intracanal instruments are made of tungsten.

   a. Both statements are true

   b. Both statements are false

   c. The first statement is true; the second statement is false.

   d. The first statement is false; the second statement is true.

5. The dentist may use several intracanal instruments beginning with a larger size and progressing to a relatively smaller size. The sizes begin with size 10 and continue in intervals of 5 to size 60.

   a. Both statements are true.

   b. Both statements are false.

   c. The first statement is true; the second statement is false.

   d. The first statement is false; the second statement is true.

6. Using the air/water syringe is not recommended for use as inside the canal, however, sodium hypochlorite can be used as an intracanal solution.

   a. Both statements are true.

   b. Both statements are false.

   c. The first statement is true; the second statement is false.

   d. The first statement is false; the second statement is true.

7. **T   F**   A glass bead sterilizer can sterilize instrument within 30 seconds depending on the type of instrument and temperature of the sterilizer.

8. The filling of the canal is primarily completed with gutta percha, though silver points can be used. Sliver points are a firm, rubber-like material that is able to precisely conform to the shape of the canal.

   a. Both statements are true.

   b. Both statements are false.

   c. The first statement is true; the second statement is false.

   d. The first statement is false; the second statement is true.

9. Irreversible pulpitis consists of lingering hot or cold sensitivity. Treatment would include a pulpotomy.

   a. Both statements are true.

   b. Both statements are false.

   c. The first statement is true; the second statement is false.

   d. The first statement is false; the second statement is true.

10. Necrotic pulp has no response on an electric or thermal pulp test. Radiographic findings include periradicular radiolucency or widened PDL.

    a. Both statements are true.

    b. Both statements are false.

    c. The first statement is true; the second statement is false.

    d. The first statement is false; the second statement is true.

CERTIFICATION REVIEW

Multiple Choice

1. Which of the following is a symptom of necrotic pulp?

   a. tooth discoloration

   b. sensitivity to cold

   c. chewing discomfort

   d. swelling

2. Which procedure uses a mild low voltage to check vitality?

   a. vitality scanner

   b. electronic pulp test

   c. thermal test

   d. percussion test

3. Which endodontic instrument is used to remove pulp tissue from the canal?

   a. paper point

   b. broach

   c. reamer

   d. gutta percha

4. Which tooth is used first when assisting during an electronic pulp pest?

   a. maxillary right central incisor

   b. mandibular left central incisor

   c. control tooth

   d. suspect tooth

5. Which instrument is usually the first instrument in the canal and barbed?

   a. reamer

   b. broach

   c. bur

   d. Hedstrom file

6. After the canal is irrigated, which is used to dry the canal?

   a. paper points

   b. gutta percha

   c. cotton pellet

   d. high-volume evacuation

7. Which of the following would be found on the tray setup for an RCT?

   a. rongeurs

   b. suture

   c. elevator

   d. Gates–Glidden drill

8. Which of the following would need to be transferred when the operator is ready to extirpate the canal?

   a. smooth broach

   b. barbed broach

   c. endodontic explorer

   d. spoon excavator

9. Which instrument would be needed during the obturation of the canal?

   a. broach

   b. file

   c. plugger

   d. high-speed handpiece

10. Which routine RCT radiograph would use the test file to find the estimated length of the canal?

    a. diagnostic

    b. trial working length

    c. working length

    d. final PA

CHAPTER APPLICATION

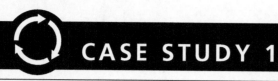

CASE STUDY 1

Jax is a 13-year-old patient who presents to the office with a deep carious lesion in tooth 31. He has not been to the dentist in quite some time, so the lesion has advanced and Jax is feeling some pain.

1. Which procedure would Jax most likely need?

_____

_____

2. Why is it important to leave some healthy pulp tissue remaining?

_____

_____

CASE STUDY 2

Sanjay comes to the office today for an emergency exam. He is feeling sensitivity in a tooth that has already been endodontically treated. After reviewing the radiograph, the endodontist decides the tooth will need to be retreated.

1. What are three reasons why an endodontically treated tooth would fail? Will Sanjay need anesthetic for the retreatment? Why or why not?

_____

_____

_____

_____

_____

_____

_____

2. What is the process of a retreatment?

_____

_____

_____

_____

Critical Thinking

1. Why is achieving adequate pain control during a root canal therapy procedure sometimes difficult?

_____

_____

_____

2. In relation to question 42, what options does the dentist have to achieve adequate pain control?

_____

_____

_____

Image Labeling

Label the following pulp tissue anatomy.

1. _____ pulp canal

2. _____ pulp chamber

3. _____ pulp horn

4. _____ pulp

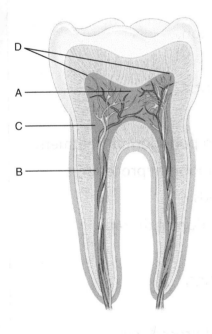

CHAPTER 38

Periodontics

At the completion of this chapter, you will be able to meet these objectives:

1. Use terms presented in this chapter.
2. Discuss the role of the members of the periodontal team.
3. Define periodontal disease.
4. Identify the causes of periodontal disease.
5. Discuss the American Association of Periodontology (AAP) classifications of periodontal disease.
6. Describe the components of the periodontal examination.
7. Describe sharpening for periodontal instruments.
8. Describe the instruments used in periodontal treatment.
9. Discuss nonsurgical methods of periodontal surgery.
10. Compare and contrast the adjunctive therapies used in periodontal treatment.
11. Discuss the healing process related to nonsurgical periodontal procedures.
12. Compare and contrast the surgical periodontal methods.
13. Outline the postoperative instructions related to periodontal therapy.
14. State the purpose of periodontal dressings.
15. Compare and contrast the types of periodontal dressings.
16. Define periodontal maintenance.
17. Describe the role of the dental assistant in periodontal procedures.

VOCABULARY BUILDER

Matching

Match each term with the appropriate definition.

1. _____ pellicle

2. _____ periodontal disease

3. _____ periodontics

4. _____ periodontium

5. _____ suppuration

6. _____ bleeding index

7. _____ periodontal probe

8. _____ curette

9. _____ periodontal knife

10. _____ periotome

a. specialty that treats the supporting tissues of the teeth and the placement, maintenance, and treatment of dental implants

b. pus in the gingival sulcus

c. a protein film that forms on the surface of the tooth

d. an instrument used to remove gingival tissue during periodontal surgery

e. is a calibrated instrument used to measure the depth of periodontal pockets, areas of recession, bleeding, or exudate

f. inflammation of the soft and hard structures that support the teeth

g. an instrument that is used to sever the periodontal ligament (PDL) prior to a traumatic extraction as well as to prepare the tissue for dental implants

h. recording the bleeding or suppuration during probing

i. tissues that support the teeth

j. a hand instrument used for removing subgingival calculus, smoothing the root surface, and removing the soft tissue lining of the periodontal pocket

CHAPTER REVIEW

Multiple Choice

1. Bacterial plaque forms around the margin of the gingiva; when left undisturbed, it mineralizes and appears as a yellow or brown deposit on the teeth called

   a. food.

   b. plaque.

   c. calculus.

   d. a stain.

2. A curved instrument is used to measure the destruction of the interradicular bone of multirooted teeth. The area where the roots divide is called the

   a. sulcus.

   b. furcation.

   c. mesiofacial.

   d. distofacial.

3. Gingival tissue is measured during the periodontal exam with a periodontal probe to evaluate

   a. plaque.

   b. calculus.

   c. mobility.

   d. recession.

4. Which hand instrument is used to remove hard deposits of supragingival and subgingival calculus from teeth? Note: The working end has two sharp edges that come to a point.

   a. scaler

   b. periodontal hoe

   c. Orban knives

   d. curette

5. Which of these are interdental knives used to remove soft tissue interproximally using long and narrow blades?

   a. Orban
   b. scalpel

   c. Kirkland
   d. pocket-marking plier

6. Which instrument is used to coagulate blood during the incising of gingival tissue?

   a. ultrasonic unit
   b. electrosurgery unit

   c. universal curette
   d. Gracey curette

7. Which instrument reflects soft tissue away from the bone?

   a. periodontal probe
   c. curette

   b. pocket-marking pliers
   d. periosteal elevator

8. The process that involves reshaping the gingival tissue to remove deformities is

   a. gingivectomy.
   b. gingivoplasty.

   c. frenectomy.
   d. mucogingival surgery.

9. Periodontal flap surgery involves surgically separating the _____ from the underlying tissue.

   a. bone
   b. tooth

   c. gingiva
   d. sulcus

10. Which procedure is a complete removal of the frenum, including the attachment to the underlying bone?

    a. frenectomy
    b. mucogingival surgery

    c. gingival grafting
    d. ostectomy

11. Periodontal probing is measuring the depth of the periodontal pocket with a periodontal probe. Each tooth will have _____ sites probed and recorded.

    a. three
    b. six

    c. two
    d. four

12. Which surgical procedure reduces the height of the gingival tissue by removing diseased gingival tissue that forms the periodontal pocket?

    a. gingivoplasty
    b. gingivectomy

    c. osteoplasty
    d. ostectomy

13. Which type of osseous surgery reshapes the bone?

    a. osteoplasty
    b. ostectomy

    c. gingivoplasty
    d. gingivectomy

14. Which type of osseous surgery removes bone?

    a. osteoplasty
    b. ostectomy

    c. gingivoplasty
    d. gingivectomy

15. A procedure in which tissue is moved from one area to another is called

    a. gingival grafting.
    b. frenectomy.

    c. flap surgery.
    d. gingivectomy.

16. What anatomical feature is characterized by a fissure or elongated opening that extends toward the root of the tooth?

    a. epithelial attachment
    b. gingival cleft

    c. sulcus
    d. periodontal ligament

17. Which evaluation method was developed by the ADA and the AAP to standardize a system of screening for periodontal disease?

    a. periodontal probing system
    b. occlusal equilibration system
    c. periodontal screening and reporting system
    d. suppuration assessment system

True or False

Circle whether the answer is true or false.

1. Diabetic patients have no greater risk of periodontal disease. These patients may have an increase in attachment and bone loss.

    a. Both statements are true.
    b. Both statements are false.
    c. The first statement is true; the second statement is false.
    d. The first statement is false; the second statement is true.

2. Stage III periodontal disease is also known as severe disease. It presents with probing depths of less than or equal to 4 mm.

    a. Both statements are true.
    b. Both statements are false.
    c. The first statement is true; the second statement is false.
    d. The first statement is false; the second statement is true.

3. Furcation involvement is noted on the periodontal chart in four different classifications according to their extent. A class III furcation involves an explorer that can pass completely through to the other side, but the gingiva is not receded.

    a. Both statements are true.
    b. Both statements are false.
    c. The first statement is true; the second statement is false.
    d. The first statement is false; the second statement is true.

4. PerioChip is a systemic antibiotic. It contains chlorhexidine gluconate.

    a. Both statements are true.
    b. Both statements are false.
    c. The first statement is true; the second statement is false.
    d. The first statement is false; the second statement is true.

5. After repeated use, the cutting edges of instruments become dull and rounded. This can cause the operator to apply more pressure, increasing operator fatigue.

    a. Both statements are true.
    b. Both statements are false.
    c. The first statement is true; the second statement is false.
    d. The first statement is false; the second statement is true.

CERTIFICATION REVIEW

Multiple Choice

1. If mixed ahead of time, which is the proper way to store a zinc oxide eugenol periodontal dressing?

   a. in the freezer
   b. in a paper towel
   c. in a cup of water
   d. in the refrigerator

2. Which instrument would be best for smoothing the root surface?

   a. curette
   b. scaler
   c. periodontal file
   d. hemostat

3. Which of the following would not be found on the gingivectomy tray setup?

   a. suture
   b. Kirkland knife
   c. scalpel handle and blade
   d. handpiece

4. Which of the following would not be found on the osseous surgery tray setup?

   a. bone file
   b. chisel scaler
   c. Kirkland knife
   d. spoon excavator

5. Following periodontal surgery, which of the following is included in the postoperative instructions?

   a. Prescription medications should be taken for 1 week following the procedure.
   b. Resume normal brushing and flossing night of surgery.
   c. Apply heat to area.
   d. Limit activity for 24 hours following surgery.

6. The operator tells you that tooth 25 has a score of 2 for mobility. How many millimeters of movement is this?

   a. 1 mm
   b. 2 mm
   c. 3 mm
   d. 4 mm

7. When the patient's tissue is described as knife-edged, this refers to which of the following?

   a. color
   b. size
   c. contour/shape
   d. consistency

8. Which periodontal instrument is spear shaped with a long narrow blade and cutting edges on both sides of the blade?

   a. Kirkland knife
   b. interdental knife
   c. Buck knife
   d. periodontal knife

9. Which periodontal instrument is used to trim tissue tags and gingival margins?

   a. periosteal elevator
   b. periodontal scissors
   c. rongeur
   d. forceps

10. The protective eyewear used during laser treatment should be cleaned with which solution?

    a. plain water
    b. soap and water
    c. Lysol
    d. isopropyl alcohol

CHAPTER APPLICATION

⟳ CASE STUDY

Joan has agreed to treatment to correct gum defects, which includes bone reshaping during surgery. Some of the damage was caused by periodontal disease.

1. What does osseous surgery involve?

_____

_____

2. What is the difference between ostectomy and osteoplasty?

_____

_____

3. What is additive osseous surgery?

_____

_____

✗ Critical Thinking

1. List the four types of periodontal dressings.

_____

_____

2. Explain why stress puts you at increased risk for periodontal disease.

_____

_____

_____

3. What are the safety procedures when using lasers?

_____

_____

_____

_____

_____

Image Labeling

1. _____ rongeurs

2. _____ periosteal elevator

3. _____ periodontal scissor

4. _____ tissue forceps

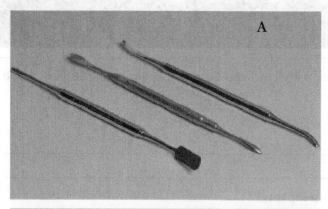

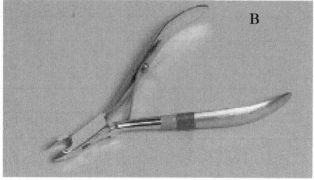

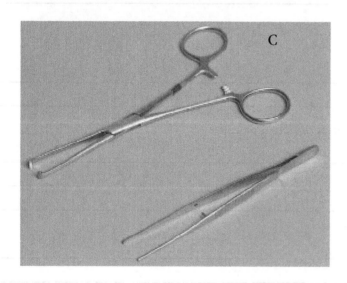

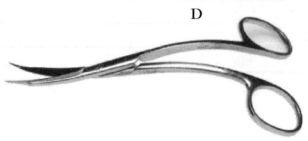

CHAPTER 39

Dental Implants

SPECIFIC INSTRUCTIONAL OBJECTIVES

At the completion of this chapter, you will be able to meet these objectives:

1. Use terms presented in this chapter.
2. State the advantages of dental implants.
3. State the disadvantages of dental implants.
4. Describe the differences in implant success rate based on location.
5. Describe the parts of an implant.
6. List the considerations for dental implants.
7. Identify the contraindications for dental implants.
8. Describe the patient selection factors for implants.
9. Describe the process for patient preparation for implant placement.
10. Compare and contrast the types of implants.
11. Describe the purpose of immediate load implants.
12. Compare and contrast the steps in the single-surgery and the two-surgery techniques.
13. Outline the postoperative home care instructions.
14. Define the implant-retained prosthesis.
15. Describe the role of the dental assistant in an implant procedure.

VOCABULARY BUILDER

Matching

Match each term with the appropriate definition.

1. _____ healing screw
2. _____ healing cap
3. _____ autograft
4. _____ allograft
5. _____ xenograft
6. _____ alloplastic graft
7. _____ surgical stent
8. _____ dysesthesia
9. _____ one-stage implant technique
10. _____ two-stage implant technique
11. _____ endosteal implant
12. _____ mini dental implant
13. _____ transosteal implant
14. _____ osteotomy
15. _____ peri-implantitis

a. grafts obtained from other human donors

b. removal of bone

c. sensation of pain

d. implant placed in bone but not covered with gingival tissue

e. template

f. also known as endosseous implant

g. inflammation of tissues surrounding implant

h. prevents growth of soft tissues over implant

i. graft from an animal source

j. offer the benefit of faster healing as compared to traditional implants

k. function as a guide for permanent restoration

l. graft harvested from patient's own body

m. grafts from synthetic materials

n. used on patients who have severely resorbed ridges

o. implant uncovered after osseointegration

True or False

Circle whether the answer is true or false.

1. **T   F**   Dental implants are one of the biggest dental advancements in the last 100 years.

2. **T   F**   The mini dental implant is smaller in diameter but wider than other implants.

3. **T   F**   The most common types of dental implants are the subperiosteal and the endosteal.

4. **T   F**   Biofilm and calculus build up on implants just like natural teeth and need to be remove routinely.

5. **T   F**   An MDI is a small metal cap that fits on a dental implant and keeps tissue and debris from getting into the implant.

6. **T   F**   Implants first became available in the 1980s.

7. **T   F**   Dental implants improve the ability to chew but do not improve esthetics.

8. **T   F**   Since dental implants do not have enamel and dentin-like natural teeth, they do not need to be maintained.

9. **T   F**   Dental implants reduce alveolar bone resorption in the edentulous area.

10. **T**   **F**   One reason an implant may fail is because the body may reject the implant.

11. **T**   **F**   The internal hex connector is shaped like an octagon.

12. **T**   **F**   Implants may be contraindicated in a patient who has a bruxism habit.

13. **T**   **F**   The endosteal implant is made of titanium.

14. **T**   **F**   Mini dental implants cost less than traditional implants.

15. **T**   **F**   It is not necessary to lay a flap for placement of a mini dental implant.

Multiple Choice

1. What is the success rate of dental implants placed in the anterior area?

   a. 80 to 100 %
   b. 90 to 100 %

   c. 85 to 95 %
   d. 75 to 85 %

2. What is the process in which a dental implant becomes fused with the bone and tissue called?

   a. orthognathic
   b. alveoplasty

   c. osseointegration
   d. a stint

3. What is the success rate of dental implants placed in the posterior area?

   a. 80 to 100 %
   b. 90 to 100 %

   c. 85 to 95 %
   d. 75 to 85 %

4. Which of the following is not a characteristic of subperiosteal implants?

   a. The dental implant is placed in the bone.

   b. They require one or two surgeries.

   c. Abutment posts are above the mucoperioseum.

   d. They are often placed with denture patients.

5. Once the dental implant is secure and stable, it holds or retains

   a. the replacement crown.
   b. the partial denture.

   c. the complete denture.
   d. all the above

CERTIFICATION REVIEW

1. How long is healing time for an implant after placement?

   a. 2 weeks
   b. 4 to 6 weeks
   c. 1 to 3 months
   d. 2 to 6 months

2. What is a contraindication for considering a patient for dental implants?

   a. Patient is in good physical health.
   b. Patient has poor oral hygiene.
   c. Patient has adequate alveolar bone.
   d. Patient has ample healing ability.

3. What is screwed into the implant and will later attach to the artificial tooth or denture?

   a. healing cap
   b. abutment post
   c. coping
   d. blade implant

4. With which of the following implants are O-rings used?

   a. endosteal
   b. periosteal
   c. transosteal
   d. mini dental implants

5. Which of the following statements about transosteal implants is not correct?

   a. They are used in the edentulous area of maxilla.
   b. They are only used with patients who have a severely absorbed alveolar ridge.
   c. These implants consist of screws, nuts, and a pressure plate.
   d. These implants are also known as staple or transosseous.

6. Which of the following statements about implant retainer prosthesis is not correct?

   a. There are two types of implant retainer prosthesis.
   b. A transitional cement is used with the cement type retainer.
   c. An amalgam restoration is placed in the crown to cover the screw.
   d. The screw retainer has two screws.

7. What type of radiographs are included in the diagnostic consultation appointment?

   a. panoramic and cephalometric
   b. bite-wing radiographs
   c. periapical radiographs
   d. occlusal radiographs

8. All of the following statements are true about the single-surgery technique *except*

   a. it involves fabricating the impression for the implant on a model.
   b. the model is constructed by using computed tomography (CT) scans.
   c. the impression is taken on the exposed alveolar bone.
   d. the implant is fabricated on the model.

9. Which of the following is/are part of the tray setup for the dental implant surgery?

   a. surgical HVE tips
   b. irrigation syringe and sterile saline solution
   c. sterile surgical drilling unit
   d. all of the above

10. In the second surgical procedure, the template is positioned and the osseointegrated implant site is marked. What is then used to excise the soft tissue and expose the healing cap of the implant?

   a. periosteal elevator
   b. electrosurgical loop
   c. surgical burs
   d. scalpel and blades

CASE STUDY

Alisha Reilly has had problems with her teeth and wants to have her mandibular teeth removed and get a denture. Her alveolar ridge has receded in the mandibular anterior area, so there is little bone to support a denture. Alisha is in good health. She is concerned about the cost, number of appointments, and how long the process will take.

1. Explain why the loss of the alveolar bone may affect the procedure.

_____
_____
_____
_____

2. Discuss her concerns about cost and the number of appointments the implant procedure may take.

_____
_____
_____
_____
_____

3. Describe why the length of time the procedure takes may vary.

_____
_____
_____
_____

Critical Thinking

1. After the dental implant procedure is completed, what is the role and responsibility of the patient to maintain the dental implant?

_____
_____
_____
_____

2. Although dental implants have a high success rate, list some of the reasons the implant may fail.

_____
_____
_____

_____

_____

_____

3. There are several techniques to the implant procedure. List the factors the dentist considers when selecting which technique to use.

_____

_____

_____

_____

_____

Fixed Prosthodontics

SPECIFIC INSTRUCTIONAL OBJECTIVES

At the completion of this chapter, you will be able to meet these objectives:

1. Use terms presented in this chapter.
2. State the objectives of fixed prosthodontics.
3. Differentiate among the types of fixed prosthodontic restorations.
4. Explain patient factors considered in a fixed prosthodontic procedure.
5. Discuss the components of the preparation appointment.
6. Paraphrase the steps in the first appointment for a fixed dental prosthesis.
7. Describe the importance of gingival retraction cord.
8. Identify the different methods of gingival retraction.
9. Discuss the process for taking an impression.
10. List the steps that take place at the lab when fabricating a fixed prosthesis.
11. Describe the communication tools available for use for communicating with the dental lab.
12. Outline the steps of the second treatment appointment for a fixed dental prosthesis.
13. Discuss the concerns related to a fixed dental prosthesis.
14. Discriminate methods of oral hygiene care for a fixed dental prosthesis.
15. Examine the changing trends related to an increase in fixed dental prosthetics.
16. Describe the components of the informed consent for fixed dental prosthodontics.
17. Identify charting symbols for a fixed prosthesis.

VOCABULARY BUILDER

Matching

Match each term with the appropriate definition.

1. _____ autoimmune
2. _____ chemotherapeutic
3. _____ crepitation
4. _____ die
5. _____ lupus
6. _____ porcelain fused to metal
7. _____ zirconia
8. _____ onlay
9. _____ inlay
10. _____ abutment
11. _____ pontic
12. _____ cantilever bridge
13. _____ Maryland bridge
14. _____ veneer
15. _____ direct resin veneer
16. _____ indirect resin veneer
17. _____ hue
18. _____ chroma
19. _____ value
20. _____ post and core

a. positive reproduction of a prepared tooth
b. part of bridge that replaces missing tooth
c. intensity of color
d. brightness of color
e. bridge retained by 1 or 2 teeth on same side
f. also known as a laminate
g. quality that differentiates colors
h. made on the patient's tooth
i. also known as a ¾ crown
j. disease that impact the skin and joints
k. replace missing tooth structure within the tooth
l. resin retained fixed bridge
m. supporting teeth of a fixed bridge
n. crackling or popping sound
o. response of an organism against itself
p. treatment of a disease with chemical agents
q. build-up of lost tooth structure
r. translucent crystalline used to make crowns
s. crown with a metal shell and porcelain cover
t. veneer that requires an impression and lab fabrication

CHAPTER REVIEW

Multiple Choice

1. Which of the following is an objective of fixed prosthodontics?

   a. restoring function
   b. improving esthetics
   c. improving speech
   d. all of the above

2. What is a prosthesis that covers the entire coronal surface of the tooth called?

   a. full crown
   b. partial crown
   c. three-quarter crown
   d. onlay

3. Which cast restoration covers the area between the cusps in the middle of the tooth, the proximal surfaces that are involved, and the cusp ridges?

   a. direct resin veneer
   b. porcelain veneer
   c. three-quarter crown
   d. porcelain fused to metal crown

4. Which restoration replaces the missing tooth structure of a mesio-occlusal surface?

   a. direct resin veneer

   b. inlay

   c. porcelain veneer

   d. porcelain fused to metal crown

5. The Maryland bridge is used to replace how many missing teeth?

   a. one

   b. two

   c. three

   d. four

6. What term describes a restoration that is composed of a thin layer of tooth-colored material that covers much of the facial surface?

   a. porcelain-fused-to-metal crowns

   b. implant-retained prostheses

   c. core buildups

   d. veneers

7. What is the name of the treatment for nonvital teeth that have very little crown structure remaining prior to placing a fixed prosthesis?

   a. veneer

   b. post and core buildup

   c. retention pin

   d. inlay

8. The dentist performs an examination to determine whether a patient is a candidate for a fixed prosthesis. Which of the following are included in this examination?

   1. exam of intraoral and extraoral tissues
   2. number of inlays
   3. radiographs
   4. retention pins
   5. diagnostic casts made
   6. implant-retained prosthesis

      a. 1, 4, 6

      b. 1, 3, 5

      c. 2, 3, 6

      d. 2, 4, 5

9. Which of the following does not take place during the first appointment for a lab-fabricated fixed prosthesis?

   a. tooth preparation

   b. final cementation of fixed prosthesis

   c. retraction cord placement around prepared tooth

   d. final impression of prepared teeth

10. Each unit of a bridge represents a tooth. The missing tooth is replaced by which of the following?

    a. pontic

    b. abutment

    c. inlay

    d. onlay

True or False

Circle whether the answer is true or false.

1. **T   F**   The retraction cord should be placed very shallowly into the sulcus so as not to injure the soft tissues.

2. **T   F**   A floss threader should be used to clean under the bridge.

3. **T   F**   Retraction cord is available as twisted or braided and comes in a variety of sizes.

4. **T   F**   Electrosurgery can be used to create a trough around the preparation if the tissues are bulbous and if esthetics are not a concern.

5. **T**   **F**   Carbide burs are used to prepare a tooth for a fixed dental prosthesis as they provide a smooth finish to the preparation.

6. **T**   **F**   The post placed into an endodontically treated tooth should be one-half the length of the root.

7. **T**   **F**   It is acceptable to use packing cord that has epinephrine as epinephrine is effective at minimizing bleeding due to its vasoconstriction effect.

8. **T**   **F**   A provisional restoration prevents the prepared tooth from fracturing or shifting while the lab is fabricating the fixed prosthesis.

9. **T**   **F**   The facebow system provides the relationship between the maxillary arch and the mandibular teeth.

10. **T**   **F**   The dental assistant may perform final cementation of the fixed prosthodontic appliance.

CERTIFICATION REVIEW

Multiple Choice

1. Which of the following is not a type of veneer?

   a. direct resin veneers
   b. indirect resin veneers
   c. direct glass ionomer veneers
   d. porcelain veneers

2. The part of the dental bridge that replaces the missing tooth is called the

   a. abutment.
   b. pontic.
   c. connector.
   d. retainer.

3. Materials used to fabricate crowns and bridges include all of the following *except*

   a. gold alloy.
   b. porcelain.
   c. acrylic.
   d. amalgam.

4. Which of the following may be the best choice on an anterior tooth when maximum esthetics is required?

   a. porcelain jacket crown
   b. porcelain fused to metal crown
   c. full gold crown
   d. nonprecious metal crown

5. Which of the following bridges is supported by an abutment on only one side?

   a. Maryland bridge
   b. cantilever bridge
   c. three unit porcelain fused to metal bridge
   d. three unit gold bridge

6. Which of the following is correct regarding a Maryland bridge?

    a. cannot be placed in areas where esthetics is a major factor

    b. can be used to replace multiple teeth

    c. has a tendency to dislodge with biting forces

    d. requires extensive tooth preparation

7. During the preparation appointment, when is the retraction cord placed?

    a. after the tooth is prepared but before the final impressions are taken

    b. after the final impressions are taken

    c. before the tooth is prepared

    d. with the provisional restoration

8. Which of the following communication tools provides information regarding the relationship between the maxilla and the temporomandibular joint?

    a. laboratory prescription form

    b. facebow transfer

    c. digital shade

    d. digital photographs

9. Which of the following is the symbol for gold in charting?

    a. Br

    b. Cl

    c. Au

    d. X

10. Which of the following is the symbol for a porcelain laminate veneer?

    a. PFM

    b. PLV

    c. Au

    d. Bll

CHAPTER APPLICATION

 # CASE STUDY 1

Because the dental assistant is involved in all stages of fixed prosthodontic treatment, understanding the sequence, preparation, and procedure is important.

1. Describe the overall sequence of dental assistant tasks during fixed prosthodontic treatment.

    _____

    _____

    _____

    _____

_____

_____

_____

_____

_____

_____

_____

_____

2. List responsibilities of the dental assistant in the preparation of equipment and supplies.

_____

_____

_____

_____

_____

_____

_____

_____

_____

_____

_____

_____

_____

_____

_____

_____

_____

_____

_____

_____

_____

3. List expanded functions related to fixed prosthodontics that may be available for assistants in certain states.

_____

_____

_____

_____

_____

_____

_____

_____

_____

_____

_____

Critical Thinking

1. Explain why the dentist may place additional retraction cords in the sulcus before the final impression is taken.

_____

_____

_____

2. Sometimes additional retention is needed during tooth preparation to improve the overall restoration. Explain when additional retention is needed, and describe the retention options.

_____

_____

_____

_____

3. What are the components of the fixed prosthodontic informed consent?

_____

_____

_____

_____

_____

_____

CHAPTER 41

Computerized Impression and Restorative Systems

SPECIFIC INSTRUCTIONAL OBJECTIVES

At the completion of this chapter, you will be able to meet these objectives:

1. Use terms presented in this chapter.

2. Explain the CAD/CAM restorative systems.

3. Compare and contrast the advantages and disadvantages of the CAD/CAM technology.

4. Explain the role of the dental assistant during CAD/CAM procedures.

5. Describe the considerations the patient should be made aware of when using CAD/CAM technology.

6. Describe the steps in a CAD/CAM procedure.

VOCABULARY BUILDER

Matching

Match each term with the appropriate definition.

1. _____ computer surface digitization

2. _____ coping

3. _____ CAD

4. _____ CAM

5. _____ digital impression system

a. involves the use of a scanner to create a digital model of the preparation

b. eliminates the need for in-office impressions

c. involves the use of a mill or special printer to fabricate the design

d. portion of a restoration made of a foundation (coping) material and a veneering material

e. used to acquire a 3D record of the geometry of the preparation in order to prepare the final restoration

CHAPTER REVIEW

Multiple Choice

1. Over the last 30 years, the CAD/CAM systems have become very popular with

   a. the fields of dentistry and endodontics.
   b. periodontics and oral maxillofacial surgery.
   c. the fields of dentistry and prosthodontics.
   d. oral maxillofacial surgery and orthodontics.

2. After the tooth is prepared:

   a. the dentist may place a retraction cord around the prepared tooth.
   b. a reflective powder may be placed to enhance the scanning process.
   c. the retraction cord is removed before the scanning begins.
   d. all of the above

3. This CAD/CAM restorative system was developed in Switzerland in 1980. It was one of the first systems on the market.

   a. iTero system
   b. Lava COS system
   c. CEREC system
   d. E4D system

4. The milling chamber contains

   a. attachment for a block of ceramic material.
   b. two diamond burs.
   c. water jet.
   d. all of the above

Matching

Match each term with the appropriate definition.

1. _____ computer-aided manufacturing (CAM)

2. _____ computer surface digitization

3. _____ CAD/CAM restorative system

4. _____ reflective powder

5. _____ digital impression system

a. becoming increasingly popular

b. Primescan

c. enhances the scanning process

d. dental laboratories use to acquire 3D record of the geometry of the preparation

e. uses software image of restoration to mill the crown, inlay, etc.

True or False

Circle whether the answer is true or false.

1. **T   F**   CAD stands for computer-advanced design.

2. **T   F**   Materials used to fabricate the restoration include all-ceramic or ceramic-resin blocks.

3. **T   F**   The second segment of the CAD/CAM system contains the intraoral camera or scanner.

4. **T   F**   The CAD/CAM system is used in both the dental office and the dental laboratory.

5. **T   F**   CEREC stands for chairside engineering restorations of esthetic ceramics.

6. **T   F**   When using the CEREC machine, there is no need to prepare the tooth first.

CERTIFICATION REVIEW

1. Which of the following types of restorations cannot be designed and milled with the CAD/CAM systems?

    a. inlays and onlays
    b. amalgam or composite
    c. posterior and anterior crowns
    d. veneers

2. All of the following are included in the tray set up for the CAD/CAM procedure *except*

    a. diamond burs and discs.
    b. slow-speed handpiece.
    c. ceramic shade guide.
    d. scaler.

3. When using a CAD/CAM system, one of the disadvantages is

    a. it does not have the ability to stain and glaze the restoration to obtain the exact shading desired by the patient and the dentist.
    b. the cost may be greater than traditional restoration procedures.
    c. the need to take additional impressions.
    d. accuracy is limited.

4. All of the following are advantages of the CAD/CAM systems *except*

    a. only one impression is taken.
    b. patient does not need to have provisional restoration.
    c. saves time for the patient.
    d. tooth sensitivity may be reduced without provisional restoration.

5. When using only a digital impression system, such as Primescan, which of the following could the patient expect when completing a restoration?

    a. returning for two visits
    b. completion in office in one visit
    c. use of alginate impressions
    d. no provisional restoration

CHAPTER APPLICATION

⟳ CASE STUDY 1

Dr. Mendoza is thinking about adding a CAD/CAM system in his office. One consideration is whether to purchase both the CAD and the CAM system or just the CAD and keep using the dental laboratory for fabricating the restorations.

1. What are the advantages of the CAD/CAM technology?

_____

_____

_____

_____

_____

_____

_____

_____

_____

_____

2. What are the disadvantages of the CAD/CAM technology?

_____

_____

_____

_____

_____

3. Describe the difference between using a CAD/CAM system versus just the CAD system.

_____

_____

_____

_____

_____

Critical Thinking

1. When the dental assistant explains to the patient the CAD/CAM option, what should be discussed?

_____

_____

2. Where is the milling machine typically located?

_____

_____

CHAPTER 42

Removable Prosthodontics

SPECIFIC INSTRUCTIONAL OBJECTIVES

At the completion of this chapter, you will be able to meet these objectives:

1. Use terms presented in this chapter.
2. Describe the objectives of removable prosthodontic treatment.
3. List the types of partial dentures.
4. Discuss the Kennedy classifications of edentulous areas.
5. Describe the types of full dentures.
6. Discuss each component of the removable partial denture (RPD).
7. Compare and contrast the indications and contraindications of RPDs.
8. Compare and contrast the advantages and disadvantages of RPDs.
9. Describe the sequence of appointments in an RPD cases.
10. Define the role of the dental assistant in an RPD case.
11. Describe each surface of the full denture.
12. Describe each component of the complete denture.
13. Compare and contrast the indications and contraindications for full dentures.
14. Compare and contrast the advantages and disadvantages of the full denture.
15. Describe the sequence of appointments in a full denture case.
16. Discuss postdelivery care related to full dentures.
17. Define the role of the dental assistant in a full denture case.
18. Explain the impact of xerostomia and its effects on the removable prosthodontic patient.
19. Explain the function of denture adhesives.
20. Compare and contrast denture relining and denture rebasing.

21. Explain the process of denture repair.

22. State the function of denture cleaners.

23. List the common abbreviations used in removable prosthodontics charting.

VOCABULARY BUILDER

Matching

Match each term with the appropriate definition.

1. _____ festooned	a. resurface the tissue side of a denture
2. _____ height of contour	b. close the margins
3. _____ peripheral seal	c. the portion of a tooth that lies between its height of contour and the gingivae.
4. _____ rebase	d. chain of material between two points
5. _____ reline	e. holes in posterior teeth areas of a denture
6. _____ undercut	f. replacement of denture saddles
7. _____ diatoric	g. highest point of a surface

Multiple Choice

1. The _____ is/are where the metal framework of the partial rests must and be prepared before the final impressions are taken.

   a. saddle
   b. border molding
   c. abutment teeth
   d. centric occlusion

2. The dental laboratory _____ the appliance on models to simulate how it will occlude and mesh in various jaw positions.

   a. relines
   b. articulates
   c. trims
   d. cleans

3. The patient moves the mouth, lips, cheeks, and tongue to establish the accurate length for the periphery and adjacent tissues to be included in the final impression. This is called _____.

   a. bite rim
   b. centric occlusion
   c. muscle trimming
   d. vertical dimension

CHAPTER REVIEW

True or False

Circle whether the answer is true or false.

1. **T F** A person is said to be edentulous when all the natural teeth are lost and no teeth remain.

2. **T   F**   A patient's posterior teeth have been extracted and dentures are constructed. Only the anterior teeth remain. Then, the anterior teeth are extracted, an alveolectomy is performed, and the denture is seated. This is called an immediate denture.

3. **T   F**   A complete denture is a type of fixed prosthesis.

4. **T   F**   Once a denture is constructed and fitted, it will be good for the life of the patient and will not require any adjustments.

5. **T   F**   The partial composed of a flexible plastic material is considered to be an esthetic option for patients.

Multiple Choice

1. Which of the following are necessary for the success of a removable dental prosthetic appliance?

   a. The patient should have a positive attitude.

   b. The patient should be cooperative.

   c. The patient should be able to maintain good oral hygiene.

   d. All of the above.

2. Which of the following is a benefit of a removable partial appliance?

   a. If a natural tooth is lost, it can be added to the partial.

   b. No oral hygiene maintenance is required.

   c. Frequent adjustment is required.

   d. All of the choices are benefits of a removable partial denture.

3. Which of the following must be determined by the dentist before treatment planning for a partial denture?

   a. The remaining teeth have adequate root structure.

   b. The patient can maintain good oral health.

   c. The alveolar bone structure is adequate.

   d. All of the above.

4. Which of the following are the parts of the removable partial denture that are positioned on the occlusal, incisal, or cingulum surfaces?

   a. connectors

   b. stress-breakers

   c. retainers

   d. rests

5. Which of the following is/are not a portion of the metal framework of a removable partial denture?

   a. rests

   b. acrylic base

   c. connectors

   d. retainers

6. Which portion of the metal framework holds the working parts in proper position?

   a. rests

   b. stress-breaker

   c. connectors

   d. clasps

7. Which portion of the partial is most often made of acrylic resin and holds the denture teeth in the dental base?

   a. stress-breaker

   b. connector

   c. retainer

   d. saddle

8. What is the acrylic material that replaces the gingival tissues in the edentulous areas?

   a. denture base

   b. bite rim

   c. vertical dimension

   d. centric occlusion

9. Which of the following surfaces of the denture is also known as the impression surface?

   a. tissue surface
   b. occlusal surface

   c. polished surface
   d. buccal surface

10. Which of the following is determined when the maxilla and the mandible are closed in a position that produces maximum contact between the occluding surfaces of the maxillary and mandibular arch?

    a. centric relation
    b. vertical dimension

    c. border molding
    d. denture base

11. When pressure from a complete or partial denture causes the supporting tissues to shrink and change in size, what procedure is used to improve the fit of the denture and comfort of the patient?

    a. overdenture
    b. try-in

    c. reline
    d. muscle trimming

12. Which of the following is a contraindication for a removable partial denture?

    a. Patient has a number of sufficiently positioned teeth in the arch.
    b. Patient has good oral home care.
    c. There is adequate root structure of the remaining teeth.
    d. There is rampant decay on existing natural teeth.

13. Which of the following provide retention of the removable partial denture away from the teeth and tissues?

    a. retainer
    b. clasp

    c. hinge
    d. connector

14. Which clasp encircles and adapts to the contours of the abutment tooth?

    a. bar
    b. circumferential

    c. retainer
    d. hinge

15. Denture borders that are too long or overextended can result in an inadequate peripheral seal. Denture borders that are too short or underextended can result in tissue changes such as epulis fissuratum.

    a. Both statements are true.
    b. Both statements are false.
    c. The first statements is true; the second statement is false.
    d. The first statements is false; the second statement is true.

CERTIFICATION REVIEW

Multiple Choice

1. Which denture appointment is the last time the dentist can make adjustments before the denture is constructed?

   a. final impressions appointment
   b. centric relation appointment
   c. oral surgery appointment
   d. try-in appointment

2. At which appointment are radiographs and preliminary impressions taken?

   a. examination and consultation appointment

   b. records appointment

   c. insertion appointment

   d. try-in appointment

3. What is the name of the device that is used to take measurements for determining the relationship of the maxillary dentition to the temporomandibular joint?

   a. facebow

   b. articulator

   c. retainer

   d. bite rims

4. Which of the following is not correct regarding the flanges of a full denture?

   a. The thickness of the labial flange provides support to the lip to improve the appearance.

   b. The buccal flange provides support to the cheeks in edentulous patients.

   c. An overextended lingual flange can cause the mandibular denture to dislodge.

   d. The post dam is the posterior edge of the mandibular denture.

5. Which of the following is defined as a Kennedy Class II?

   a. The edentulous area is unilateral and is located posterior to the remaining natural teeth.

   b. The edentulous area is unilateral with natural teeth remaining anterior and posterior to it.

   c. The edentulous areas are bilateral and are located posterior to the remaining natural teeth.

   d. The edentulous area is a single, bilateral area that crosses the midline located anterior to the remaining natural teeth.

6. Your patient presents for a try-in visit of a full denture. Which of the following statement is correct about the try-in visit?

   a. The wax rims are present on the denture base.

   b. The teeth are present on the try-in appliance.

   c. The shade selection will be completed at the try-in visit.

   d. The initial centric relation will be obtained at the try-in visit.

7. In the construction of complete dentures, which of the following visits follows the final try-in visit?

   a. obtaining centric relation

   b. obtaining the shade

   c. try-in of wax rims on baseplates

   d. insertion of the finished denture

8. Which of the following instruments should be included on the tray setup for the try-in visit of full dentures?

   a. processed and finished final full dentures

   b. facebow

   c. bite registration material

   d. articulating paper

9. Which of the following instruments is not needed on the tray setup for a chairside denture reline?

    a. articulating paper
    b. reline material
    c. pressure indicator paste
    d. cotton rolls

10. Which of the following is correct regarding full dentures?

    a. It is easier for patients to adapt to a mandibular full denture as opposed to a maxillary full denture.
    b. The mandibular denture has suction for retention whereas the maxillary denture does not.
    c. The denture base disperses the forces on the teeth and the tissues.
    d. Gold is a commonly used material today for denture bases.

CHAPTER APPLICATION

 CASE STUDY 1

After a recent luncheon with friends, during which she was anxious about her denture becoming loose, Rachel decided that she needed to consult with her dentist. Following an examination, the dentist recommended a denture reline.

1. How will the reline benefit Rachel?

2. What are the benefits of a soft reline?

3. What is the difference between a laboratory reline and a chairside reline?

CASE STUDY 2

The dental assistant's functions include recording measurements and details for the fabrication of the denture, as well as providing education and support to patients. Ester is coming in for a detailed examination in preparation for a complete denture.

1. What features are examined during an intraoral cavity examination?

   _____

   _____

   _____

   _____

   _____

2. In addition to the results of the intraoral examination, list other supportive documentation that will assist in the overall evaluation.

   _____

   _____

   _____

3. Describe the use of past photographs as a diagnostic tool.

   _____

   _____

   _____

   _____

4. List the types of data collected and used in devising the final treatment plan.

   _____

   _____

   _____

   _____

   _____

   _____

X Critical Thinking

1. Fred will receive a full maxillary denture. Because he still has anterior teeth and is concerned about going without any teeth while continuing to work, he selected an immediate denture procedure. Explain how the baseplate, rim, and occlusal relationship measurements are taken.

   _____

   _____

   _____

   _____

_____

_____

_____

2. A sequence of appointments helps the patient and the dental assistant to be ready for each step of the process. List the suggested series of appointments for a complete denture.

_____

_____

_____

_____

_____

_____

_____

_____

_____

_____

_____

_____

_____

_____

_____

_____

_____

_____

CHAPTER 43

Cosmetic Dentistry and Teeth Whitening

At the completion of this chapter, you will be able to meet these objectives:

1. Use terms presented in this chapter.
2. Describe the duties and credentialing of the cosmetic dental team.
3. Discuss procedures that are included in cosmetic dentistry.
4. Explain how teeth are whitened.
5. Discuss indications in selecting candidates for dental whitening.
6. Discuss contraindications in selecting candidates for dental whitening.
7. Describe the procedures for dental office whitening for vital and nonvital teeth.
8. Describe the procedures for home whitening and over-the-counter whitening materials.
9. Discuss esthetic prostheses that are used in cosmetic dentistry.
10. Discuss the role of occlusion in cosmetic dentistry.
11. Discuss the role of contouring soft tissues in cosmetic dentistry.

VOCABULARY BUILDER

Matching

Match each term with the appropriate definition.

1. _____ vertical dimension of occlusion

   a. the science of occlusion that objectively measures the physiologic functions affected by occlusion to achieve an optimal relationship between the skull and the mandible

2. _____ neuromuscular dentistry

3. _____ hydrogen peroxide

4. _____ carbomide peroxide

5. _____ sodium perborate

b. the distance between the maxilla and the mandible when the teeth are in full occlusion

c. a weak oxidizing agent which is used to whiten nonvital teeth

d. varies in strength from a 5 to 35% solution and breaks down into water and oxygen

e. a complex form of urea and hydrogen peroxide which varies in strength from a 10 to 20% solution

Fill in the Blank

Please fill in the blank with one of the choices provided.

(bleaching, whitening; lightening, bleaching; whitening, lightening; whitening, bleaching)

1. The term _____ refers to the restoration of a tooth's surface by removing dirt and debris. The term _____ to be used only when the teeth can be whitened beyond their natural color.

CHAPTER REVIEW

Multiple Choice

1. The _____ is the largest dental organization dedicated to the art and science of cosmetic dentistry.

   a. ADA

   b. AACD

   c. OTC

   d. CD

2. Gingival tissue enlargement may make the teeth appear shorter than normal. What procedure could be performed to improve the appearance of a patient with this condition?

   a. crown lengthening

   b. placement of veneers

   c. soft tissue contouring

   d. gingival grafting

3. Whitening agents used in toothpaste include

   a. hydrogen peroxide.

   b. sodium bicarbonate.

   c. aluminum trihydroxide.

   d. none of the above

4. All of the following are OTC whitening products except

   a. strips.

   b. chewing gum.

   c. composite resin.

   d. toothpaste.

5. All of the following are commonly used whitening agents except

   a. sodium perborate.

   b. sodium bicarbonate.

   c. hydrogen peroxide.

   d. carbamide peroxide

6. What type of teeth is power whitening performed on

   a. nonvital

   b. vital

   c. endodontic

   d. none of the above

7. Which whitening is used to lighten an endodontically treated tooth.

   a. walking

   b. assisted

   c. OTC

   d. power

8. Which of the following documentation activities would be included as part of routine procedure for all cosmetic dentistry treatments?

   a. Document that a conclusive treatment plan was given to the patient, and a consent form was signed before treatment began.

   b. Document any adverse occurrences or problems that arose during the course of treatment.

   c. Document instances when the patient did not follow home-care instructions.

   d. all of the above

9. When restoring anterior teeth, which of the following can be used to restore shade, length, and shape of an anterior tooth or teeth?

   a. veneer

   b. removable partial denture

   c. implant

   d. denture

True or False

Circle whether the answer is true or false.

1. **T   F**   Cosmetic dentistry is a recognized specialty of dentistry by the American Dental Association.

2. As a fellowship in the American Academy of Cosmetic Dentistry, the dentist must take continuing education courses and pass an examination process. An accredited member submits 50 clinical cases that exhibit competency in cosmetic dentistry.

   a. Both statements are true.

   b. Both statements are false.

   c. The first statement is true, the second statement is false.

   d. The first statement is false, the second statement is true.

CERTIFICATION REVIEW

Multiple Choice

1. Which of the following is an indication for tooth whitening?

   a. color change related to pulpal trauma and necrosis

   b. pregnancy

   c. hypersensitive teeth

   d. discoloration caused by tetracycline

2. How many millimeters of gingiva should be visible in a normal smile?

   a. 1–2 mm

   b. 2–4 mm

   c. 4–6 mm

   d. 6+ mm

3. For an in-office whitening procedure on vital teeth, which is performed first?

   a. polishing the crowns of the teeth

   b. recording a shade

   c. placement of dental dam

   d. placing on barrier gel

4. Which is an advantage of in-office whitening?

   a. less cost to patient

   b. quick and noticeable color change in short period of time

   c. can vary percentage and duration based on sensitivity

   d. less sensitivity

5. When setting up for an in-office whitening procedure on vital teeth, which of the following should be included on the tray?

   a. high-speed handpiece

   b. high-volume evacuation

   c. UV curing light

   d. scaler

6. Which of the following can be side effects of OTC whitening materials?

   a. temporary tooth sensitivity

   b. temporary gingival sensitivity

   c. irreversible tooth damage

   d. all of the above

7. When grafting tissue, tissue is taken from which area of the mouth?

   a. soft palate

   b. hard palate

   c. buccal mucosa

   d. labial mucosa

CHAPTER APPLICATION

Critical Thinking

1. Describe how teeth are whitened.

   _____

   _____

   _____

   _____

2. Explain the difference between extrinsic and intrinsic stains.

   _____

   _____

   _____

3. What are the advantages and disadvantages of take home office assistant whitening?

   _____

   _____

   _____

   _____

4. When taking a shade before whitening, why should the teeth not be dried?

   _____

   _____

5. Describe how chewing gum whitening works.

   _____

   _____

   _____

6. Placing cosmetic restorations has a significant impact on occlusion. Why?

_____

_____

_____

⟳ CASE STUDY

Maria comes to the office with #8 being nonvital. There is some darker staining beginning on the tooth and Maria is concerned. She is in today to see her options for lightening this tooth.

1. Why did Maria's tooth turn dark?

_____

_____

_____

2. What are the two options Maria can choose from?

_____

_____

3. Describe each technique.

_____

_____

_____

_____

_____

_____

_____

_____

Dental Practice Management

Dental Practice Management

SPECIFIC INSTRUCTIONAL OBJECTIVES

At the completion of this chapter, you will be able to meet these objectives:

1. Use terms presented in this chapter.
2. Explain the appropriate format of a welcome letter.
3. Identify marketing ideas for dentistry.
4. Identify the components of a reception area.
5. Identify the dental office staff and their areas of responsibility.
6. Outline the proper procedure for answering an incoming call.
7. Describe proper phone messaging etiquette.
8. Describe telephone and business office technology and its uses.
9. Discuss the presentation of a patient care plan.
10. Explain the different elements that go into appointment scheduling.
11. Compare and contrast a computerized recare system to a manual recare system.
12. Give examples of the ways in which computers are used in the dental office.
13. Differentiate between expendable and nonexpendable supplies.
14. Explain why ergonomics is important at a computer workstation.
15. Describe the use of a computerized inventory management system.
16. Identify computerized and manual systems for the management of patient accounts.
17. Discuss the different aspects of managing office finances.
18. Explain dental insurance as it applies to the dental office.
19. List common examples of insurance fraud made by dental practices.
20. Explain common dental benefit and claim terminology.
21. Discuss common avenues of teledentistry.

VOCABULARY BUILDER

Matching

Match each term with the appropriate definition.

1. _____ asynchronous	a. the ability to change in size
2. _____ capitation	b. amount due for services submitted to the insurer or patient
3. _____ claim	c. scheduled payment for providing services to patients who either choose or are assigned to the practice
4. _____ proprietary	d. communication that is pre-recorded and not occurring at the same time
5. _____ scalability	e. having ownership

Fill in the Blank

Please fill in the blank with one of the choices provided.

(allowances, semiblock, full block, Time block, proprietary, a lifetime, capitation, disposable)

1. The maximum benefit of a health plan will pay to an insured individual is calculated over _____.

2. A business letter with all information justified against the left margin is a _____.

3. Products that are designed for being thrown away are _____ supplies.

4. _____ is a block in the schedule for a time of the day for use other than procedures.

5. A sum of money allotted or granted for a particular purpose, such as expenses, is _____.

CHAPTER REVIEW

Multiple Choice

1. Which accounting term indicates the money owed to a practice?

   a. accounts payable
   b. accounts receivable
   c. inventory
   d. nonexpendable

2. Which accounting term indicates the amount a practice owes to others?

   a. gross income
   b. accounts payable
   c. accounts receivable
   d. petty cash

3. Which of the following items is not part of a computer function?

   a. spreadsheet
   b. word processing
   c. cellular phone
   d. database management

4. The goal of the receptionist is to fill the appointment book with patient care. Any time in the appointment book that is not scheduled is called:

a. downtime.

b. overtime.

c. overlap time.

d. tickler file.

5. When you subtract the accounts payable from gross income, the result is the:

a. overhead.

b. net income.

c. gross income.

d. petty cash.

6. There are several inventory record systems that can be used to track supplies. Supplies that are retained in the office for long periods of time are called:

a. nonexpendable.

b. expendable.

c. shelf life.

d. variable.

7. Which of the following are basic telephone techniques?

1. Enunciate, speak clearly, and articulate carefully.
2. State who the message is for.
3. Speak at a normal rate of speed.
4. Ask what action is required.
5. Use telephone etiquette (good manners, avoid slang).
6. Record the date and time of the call.

a. 1, 2, 6

b. 1, 3, 6

c. 1, 3, 5

d. 1, 4, 6

8. As part of the office's business equipment, answering systems may include which of the following features?

1. voice mail
2. e-mail
3. word processing
4. fax
5. graphics
6. database management

a. 3, 4, 6

b. 1, 2, 6

c. 2, 3, 4

d. 1, 2, 4

9. _____ requires that the sender receives a confirmation of delivery.

a. collect on delivery

b. delivery confirmation

c. insured mail

d. certified mail

10. Total accounts receivable are calculated as _____ income.

a. gross

b. net

c. deductible

d. expendable

True or False

Circle whether the answer is true or false.

1. As health care workers, we are responsible to try and meet the needs of all patients, including those with language barriers. It is not always feasible to have supply an interpreter, so a patient may bring family member who can translate.

    a. Both statements are true.

    b. Both statements are false.

    c. The first statement is true; the second statement is false.

    d. The first statement is false; the second statement is true.

2. **T   F**   In order to safeguard a fax machine, do not leave any forms in machine after facsimile is transmitted.

3. **T   F**   When scheduling an appointment for a child, it is best to remember the child is at their best in the afternoon.

4. **T   F**   Graphics software is a program that allows numerical data to be analyzed.

5. When designing the schedule, block out times for higher production. About 30% of your production should be completed in the morning.

    a. Both statements are true.

    b. Both statements are false

    c. The first statement is true; the second statement is false.

    d. The first statement is false; the second statement is true.

6. A computer hardware is the computer's physical equipment, and the software is a computer program or set of instructions.

    a. Both statements are true.

    b. Both statements are false.

    c. The first statement is true; the second statement is false.

    d. The first statement is false; the second statement is true.

Matching

Inventory control is effective when using an expendable and nonexpendable inventory supply system. Match each term with its description.

Term	Description
1. _____ price break	a. length of time that product can be stored
2. _____ rate of use	b. ensures that adequate supply is available
3. _____ reorder point	c. how much product is used in a specific period
4. _____ shelf life	d. minimum quantity of supply at which the per unit cost is reduced

CERTIFICATION REVIEW

Multiple Choice

1. What are the codes which are used for dental insurance purposes, are published under the jurisdiction of the American Dental Association.

   a. COD

   b. USPS

   c. CDT

   d. TDI

2. Composite material is classified as a/an

   a. consumable supply.

   b. disposable supply.

   c. expendable.

   d. major equipment.

3. A fee schedule is used to define what patients will be charged for a particular service. This is called the

   a. professional courtesy.

   b. usual, reasonable, and customary fee.

   c. insurance.

   d. record management.

4. Which of the following is not a component of a letter?

   a. inside address

   b. outside address

   c. salutation

   d. date

5. When recording an away message for the office, what should be included?

   a. the doctor's home phone number

   b. where the nearest hospital is

   c. the reason the office is closed

   d. the address of the office

6. What is the most secure type of mail, which ensures the protection of important mail?

   a. certified

   b. insured

   c. registered

   d. priority

7. The insurance deductible is which of the following?

   a. the amount paid before benefits take effect

   b. determination of whether a patient is eligible for dental benefits

   c. a payment made by the carrier to the patient

   d. the amount the carrier charges the subscriber

8. Which of the following is true of semiblock letters?

   a. all left justified

   b. double spaced

   c. indentation of each paragraph

   d. all right justified

9. Blocks of time set aside for emergency patients are called

   a. double booking.

   b. buffer time.

   c. down time.

   d. overlap time.

10. To authorize direct pay to the provider, what portion of an insurance form requires the patient's signature?

    a. eligibility

    b. informed consent

    c. beneficiary

    d. assignment of benefits

CHAPTER APPLICATION

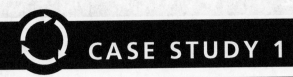

CASE STUDY 1

Accurate dental record management is essential for quality patient care in any dental office. Patients have the right to expect confidential treatment and record-keeping.

1. Describe equipment and supplies needed for record management.

   _____

   _____

2. Describe the patient chart filing system.

   _____

   _____

   _____

3. Explain the record confidentiality policy.

   _____

   _____

   _____

   _____

   _____

   _____

4. Describe archival storage of records.

   _____

   _____

   _____

   _____

   _____

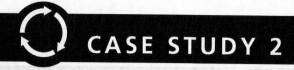

CASE STUDY 2

Some patients will experience financial difficulties. The dentist must provide guidelines for business office employees on when and how to contact patients with past-due accounts.

1. List four tips for collections by telephone.

_____

_____

_____

_____

_____

_____

_____

_____

_____

_____

_____

_____

2. Describe when a collection agency would be used.

_____

_____

3. Explain when collection letters are initiated.

_____

_____

Critical Thinking

1. Dental coverage and benefits available to patients become more complex over time. Describe indemnity plans and capitation programs.

_____

_____

_____

_____

_____

2. An understanding of dental insurance terminology is critical when filing claims. Explain the difference between explanation of benefits (EOB) and coordination of benefits (COB).

_____

_____

_____

_____

3. Explain what the birthday rule is.

_____

_____

_____

_____

Career Planning

SPECIFIC INSTRUCTIONAL OBJECTIVES

At the completion of this chapter, you will be able to meet these objectives:

1. Use terms presented in this chapter.
2. Research the state credentialing requirements.
3. Develop personal career objective.
4. Create personal career portfolio.
5. Compose master electronic cover letter and résumé.
6. Request references for letter of recommendations.
7. List ways a job seeker can begin a job search.
8. Discuss arranging for an interview.
9. Complete job application accurately and thoroughly.
10. Prepare for preinterview.
11. Describe how to interview for dental assisting position.
12. Describe the goal of job orientation of a new employee.
13. Explain what the employee can do to keep their job.
14. Explain how to handle being placed on performance or professional probation and being fired.
15. Develop plan for career and job advancement.
16. Defend the need for professional development and continuing education.

VOCABULARY BUILDER

Matching

Match each term with the appropriate definition.

1. _____ portfolio
2. _____ cover letter
3. _____ header
4. _____ salutation
5. _____ résumé
6. _____ reference
7. _____ networking
8. _____ interview
9. _____ application
10. _____ probation

a. addresses recipient

b. personal connections to find a job

c. identifies areas where employee needs to improve

d. letter of introduction

e. brief account of qualifications

f. formal meeting with employer

g. assistant's personal contact information

h. person to vouch for qualifications

i. form used to learn facts about applicant

j. showcases the assistant's best work

CHAPTER REVIEW

True or False

Circle whether the answer is true or false.

1. **T F** A portfolio is a collection of evidence to showcase your best work at an interview.

2. **T F** The best job references to include with your résumé are previous teachers, past employers, and family members.

3. **T F** It is better to address your cover letter as "Dear Employer" instead of directly addressing the dentist by name.

4. **T F** When addressing the dentist in the recipient information section of a cover letter, it should be written as "Dr. John Smith, D. D. S."

5. **T F** When addressing the dentist in the salutation section of a cover letter, it should be written as "Dear Doctor Smith."

6. **T F** A résumé and letter of recommendations are often included as enclosures in a cover letter.

7. **T F** It is important to get a reference's permission and to inform them of your most recent accomplishments to prepare them for a call from a potential employer.

8. **T F** It is helpful to include letters of recommendations in your job portfolio.

Multiple Choice

1. In developing a cover letter, there is a standard format that follows a specific order. Place the following items in the order in which they would appear in a cover letter.

   1. salutation
   2. header

    3. enclosures

    4. recipient information

    5. closing

    6. body of letter

      a. 1, 2, 4, 6, 3, 5

      b. 2, 4, 1, 6, 5, 3

      c. 1, 2, 3, 4, 5, 6

      d. 2, 1, 4, 6, 5, 3

2. The résumé should fit on a single page and follow the standard format. Place the following items in the order in which they would appear in a résumé.

    1. education

    2. work experience

    3. career objective

    4. identification

    5. references

    6. activities

      a. 3, 4, 1, 2, 6, 5

      b. 3, 4, 2, 1, 5, 6

      c. 4, 3, 1, 2, 6, 5

      d. 4, 3, 2, 1, 5, 6

3. When preparing for the interview, there are several things to think about. Which of the following items make for a successful interview?

    1. Arrive 5 minutes early.

    2. Wear jeans.

    3. Smile.

    4. Demonstrate good hygiene.

    5. Control the interview.

    6. Be a good speller.

      a. 1, 3, 5

      b. 1, 3, 4

      c. 3, 4, 6

      d. 3, 4, 5

4. As an employee in a health profession, maintaining high standards includes

    a. personal hygiene.

    b. clean uniforms.

    c. clean shoes.

    d. all of the above

5. If the dentist requires a working interview, what can you do to have a successful interview?

    a. Ask about responsibilities for the day.

    b. Ask pertinent questions.

    c. Ask if there is anything you can do during downtimes.

    d. all of the above

6. When salary has not been mentioned throughout the interviewing process, when should it be discussed?

    a. when setting up the interview

    b. after receiving the employment offer

    c. during the interview

    d. both a. and b.

7. Which of the following elements should be covered in a practice interview?

    a. Offer handshake at the end of the interview.

    c. Tell stories that support your answers.

    b. Make eye contact.

    d. all of the above

8. Personal appearance influences perceptions during the interviewing process. All of the following are recommended EXCEPT

    a. Demonstrate good hygiene.

    b. Dress casually.

    c. Remove piercings.

    d. Lightly apply cologne.

9. All of the following are requirements for keeping a job EXCEPT:

   a. Always look professional.

   b. Be well prepared for the job.

   c. Always be on time.

   d. Blame other staff members when you make a mistake.

10. Any number of dentists (both general and specialty) can share a building and still remain independent. This type of dental office is called a:

    a. specialty practice.

    b. partnership.

    c. group practice.

    d. solo practice.

11. A dentist may hire another dentist under a contractual agreement. This hired dentist is called a dental:

    a. partner.

    b. solo.

    c. associate.

    d. group.

12. In (a/an) _____, the dental assistant treats patients who are eligible to receive dental care at a reduced rate.

    a. group practice

    b. government clinic

    c. solo practice

    d. insurance programmer

13. To obtain employment in a _____ facility, the dental assistant must obtain employment through the civil service.

    a. federal

    b. state

    c. dental school

    d. veterans' hospital

14. Qualities that a dentist looks for in a dental assistant include which of the following?

    a. good clinical skills

    b. team player

    c. good interpersonal skills

    d. all of the above

CERTIFICATION REVIEW

Multiple Choice

1. What should the dental assistant read to determine which duties they can legally perform?

   a. DANB outline

   b. federal dental practice act

   c. state dental practice act

   d. state board of health

2. To terminate employment in your office, how much notice should you provide your employer?

   a. one month

   b. two weeks

   c. one week

   d. two days

3. Eligibility for national certification can be obtained by which of the following criteria for Pathway I?

   1. high school graduation or equivalent

   2. current CPR card from a DANB-accepted CPR provider

   3. verification of dentist employer

   4. graduation from an accredited dental assistant or dental hygiene program

5. six months full-time employment

6. 3,500 hours of employment

    a. 1, 6

    b. 2, 5

    c. 2, 4

    d. 1, 5

4. National certification for dental assistants is not mandatory in every state. The _____ assumes the responsibility for credentialing dental assistants.

    a. ADAA

    b. DANB

    c. ADA

    d. AMA

5. If job performance expectations and/or responsibilities are unclear, which should the dental assistant refer to for clarification?

    a. Observe procedures being performed.

    b. Ask an experienced dental assistant.

    c. Read the office procedure manual.

    d. all of these

CHAPTER APPLICATION

 CASE STUDY 1

Phoebe is excited but anxious about an upcoming interview. In preparation for the interview, she began listing things to do.

1. List items to consider when preparing for an interview.

    _____

    _____

2. Explain the types of questions that can be asked by the applicant during an interview and those that should be avoided.

    _____

    _____

    _____

3. Describe the mock interview.

    _____

    _____

4. Describe appropriate attire for an interview.

    _____

Critical Thinking

Answers for these critical thinking questions are based on the student's personal response—there is not a correct response, and answers should be evaluated on acceptable response.

1. One of the first steps you should complete before seeking your first job is to form your career objective. Your career objective should include what you want. Answer the following questions to help you focus on what you want.

   a. What position do you want?

   b. What do you want to do?

   c. Where do you want to work?

2. You may be required to complete a job application at the time of the interview. Coming with a completed data sheet will show that you are conscientious and prepared. Complete the following data sheet for your interviews.

Applicant's Name (Last)	First	Middle Initial	Social Security Number - -
Mailing Address (Number)	Street		Work Telephone Number ( )
City	State	Zip Code	Home Telephone Number ( )

EDUCATION

Name of School	Location of School	Degree or Course of Study	Date Completed

EMPLOYMENT HISTORY – Begin with your most recent job. List each job separately.

Job Title	Dates Worked From _____ To _____	Pay $ _____ Per _____
Name of Employer	Name of Supervisor	
Address:	City State Zip Code	
Telephone Number ( )	Reason for Leaving:	
Duties Performed:		

Job Title	Dates Worked From _____ To _____	Pay $ _____ Per _____
Name of Employer	Name of Supervisor	
Address:	City State Zip Code	
Telephone Number ( )	Reason for Leaving:	
Duties Performed:		

Job Title		Dates Worked From _____ To _____		Pay $ _____ Per _____
Name of Employer			Name of Supervisor	
Address:	City		State	Zip Code
Telephone Number ( )		Reason for Leaving:		
Duties Performed:				

Job Title		Dates Worked From _____ To _____		Pay $ _____ Per _____
Name of Employer			Name of Supervisor	
Address:	City		State	Zip Code
Telephone Number ( )		Reason for Leaving:		
Duties Performed:				

PERSONAL REFERENCES: List the names of three references that employers may contact.

1) Name	Telephone # ( )	Relationship (Teacher etc.)
Address:	City	State	Zip Code

2) Name	Telephone # ( )	Relationship (Teacher etc.)
Address:	City	State	Zip Code

3) Name	Telephone # ( )	Relationship (Teacher etc.)
Address:	City	State	Zip Code

3. Practicing common interview questions helps prepare you for a successful interview.

   Answer the following questions:

   a. Why did you become a dental assistant?

   b. Why do you want this position?

   c. What does teamwork mean to you? Are you a team player?

   d. Can you deal with a lot of different types of people all day?

   e. Do you work well under stress?

   f. What do you see yourself doing in five years?

   g. Why do you want to work here?

   h. How would you describe the value of a dental treatment to a patient?

   i. What is the most important aspect of a successful dental practice?

   j. What do you think are the most important attributes of a dental assistant?

   k. What are your strengths as a dental assistant?

   l. What are your weaknesses as a dental assistant?

   m. Explain four handed dentistry.

   n. What will you bring to my practice to increase productivity and revenue?

   o. What type of patient do you like to work with, and what ones you do not like to work with?

Notes

Notes

Notes

Notes

Notes

Notes

Notes

Notes

Notes

Notes

Notes

Notes